# Butterflies

## PICTURE BOOK

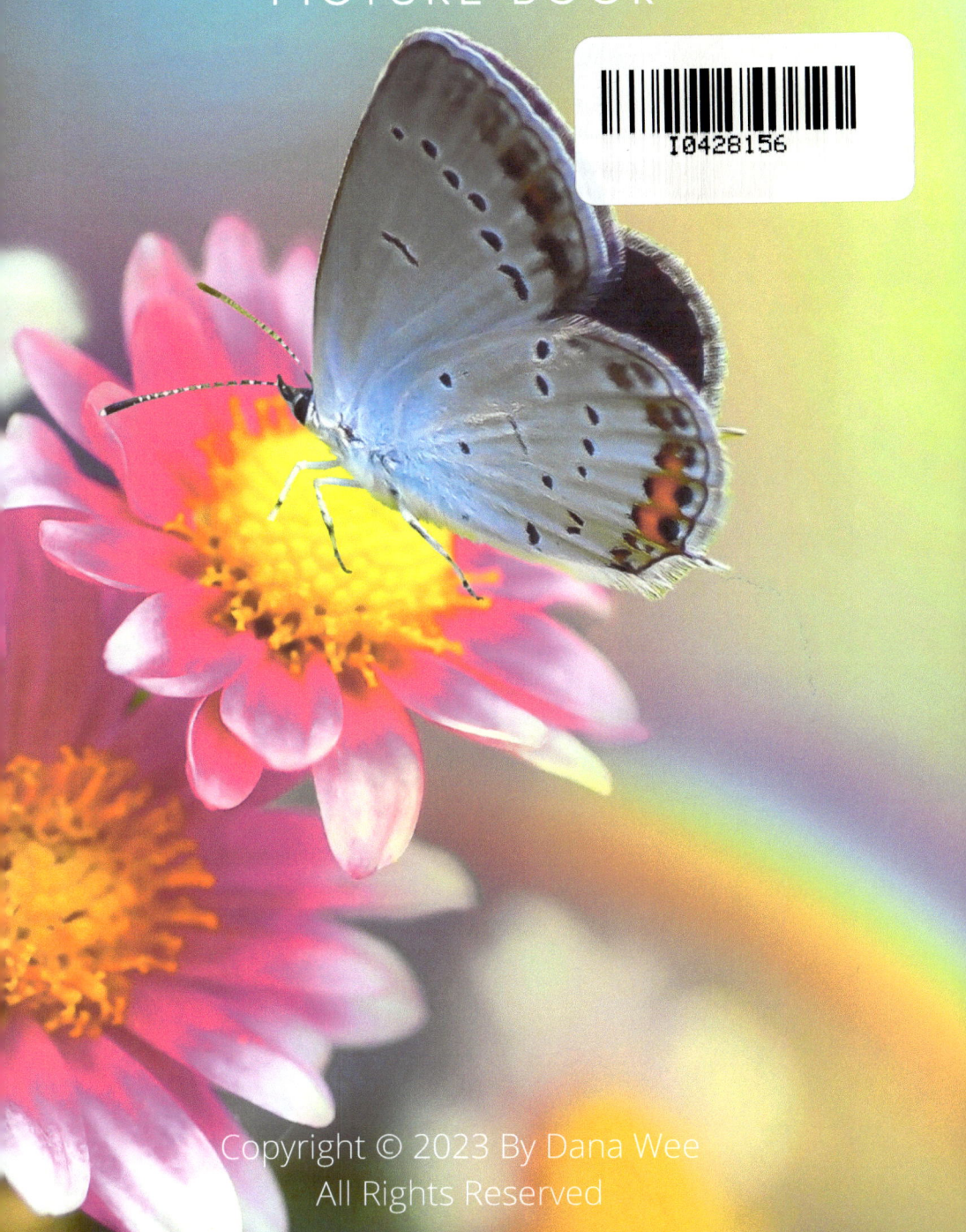

I0428156

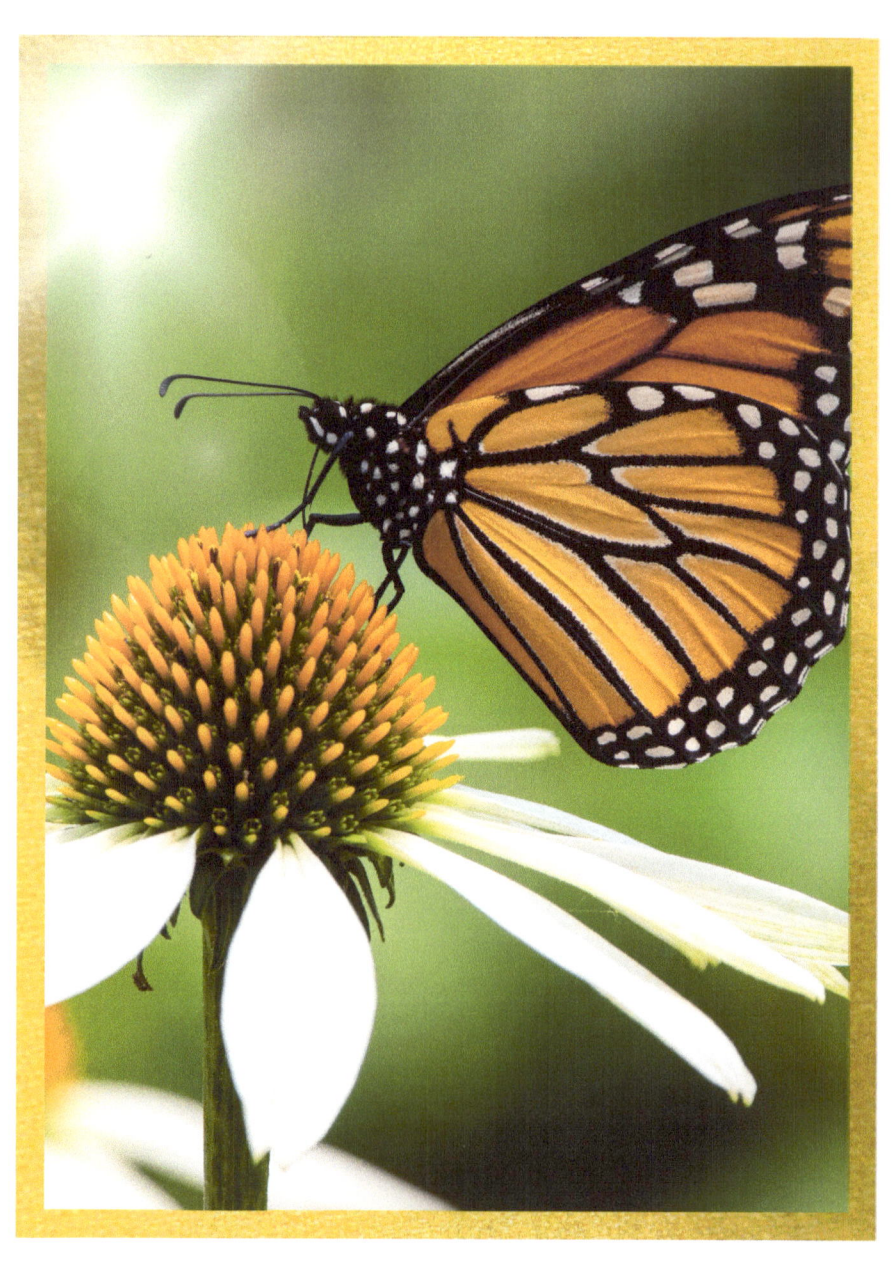

Good morning!
Time to work

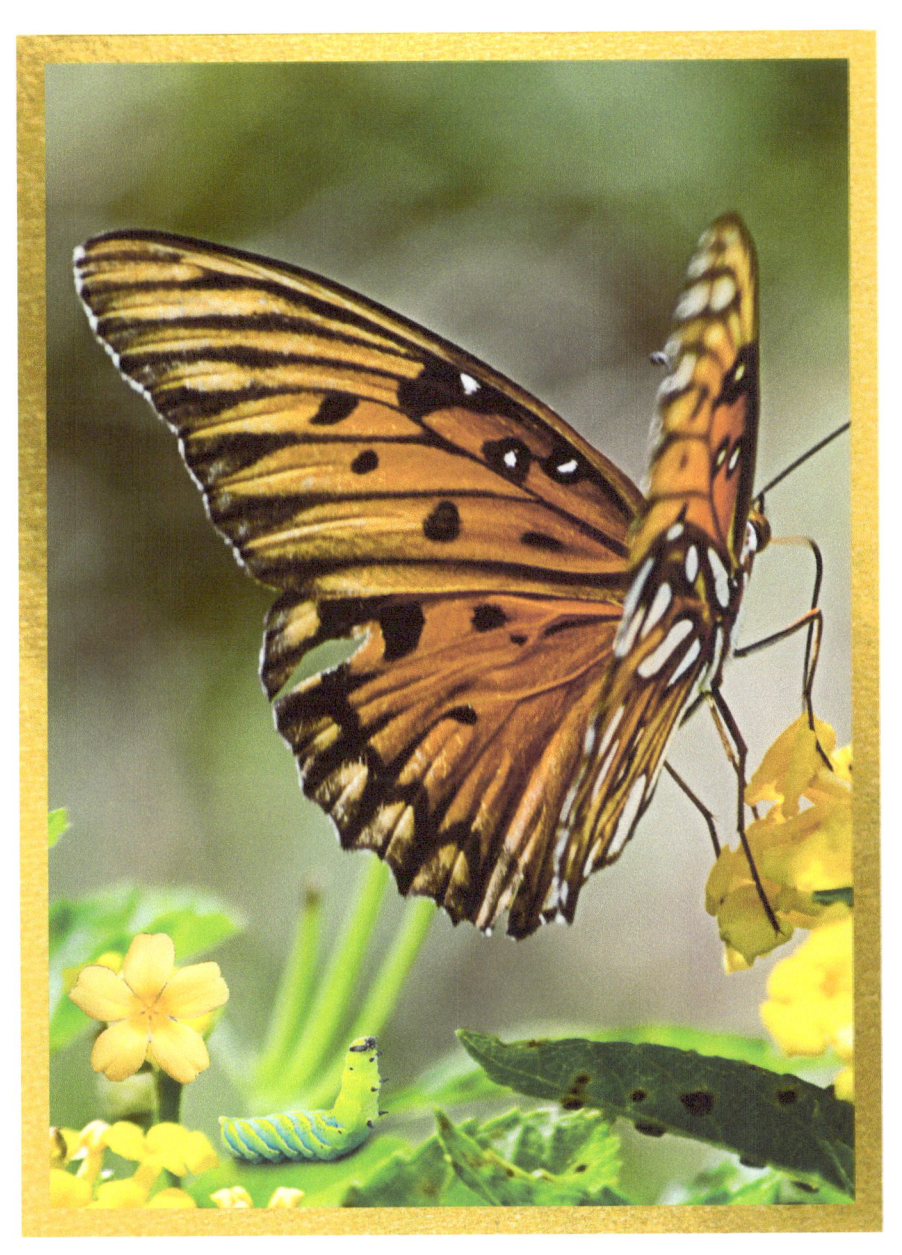

Nature in it's own natural beauty

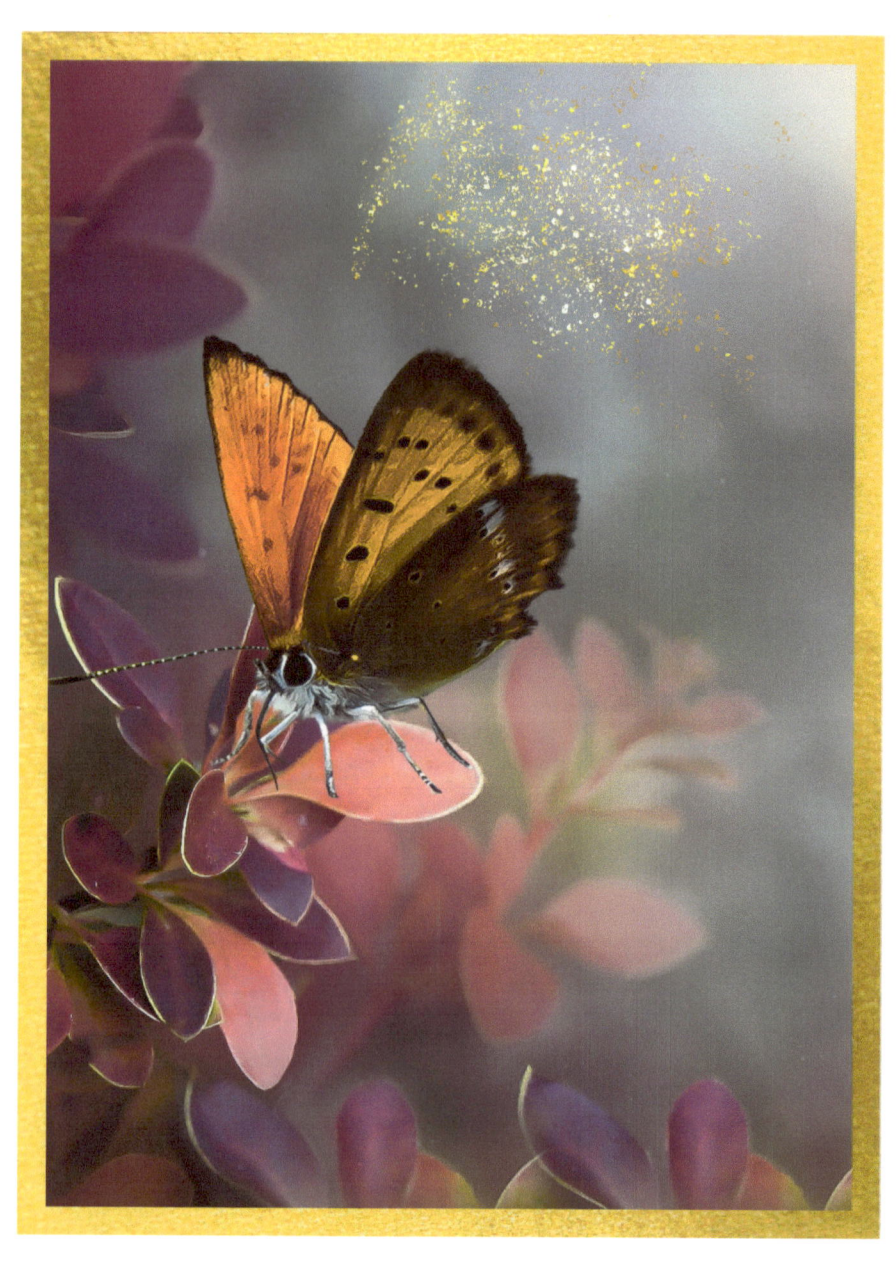

Rare gem on a misty morning

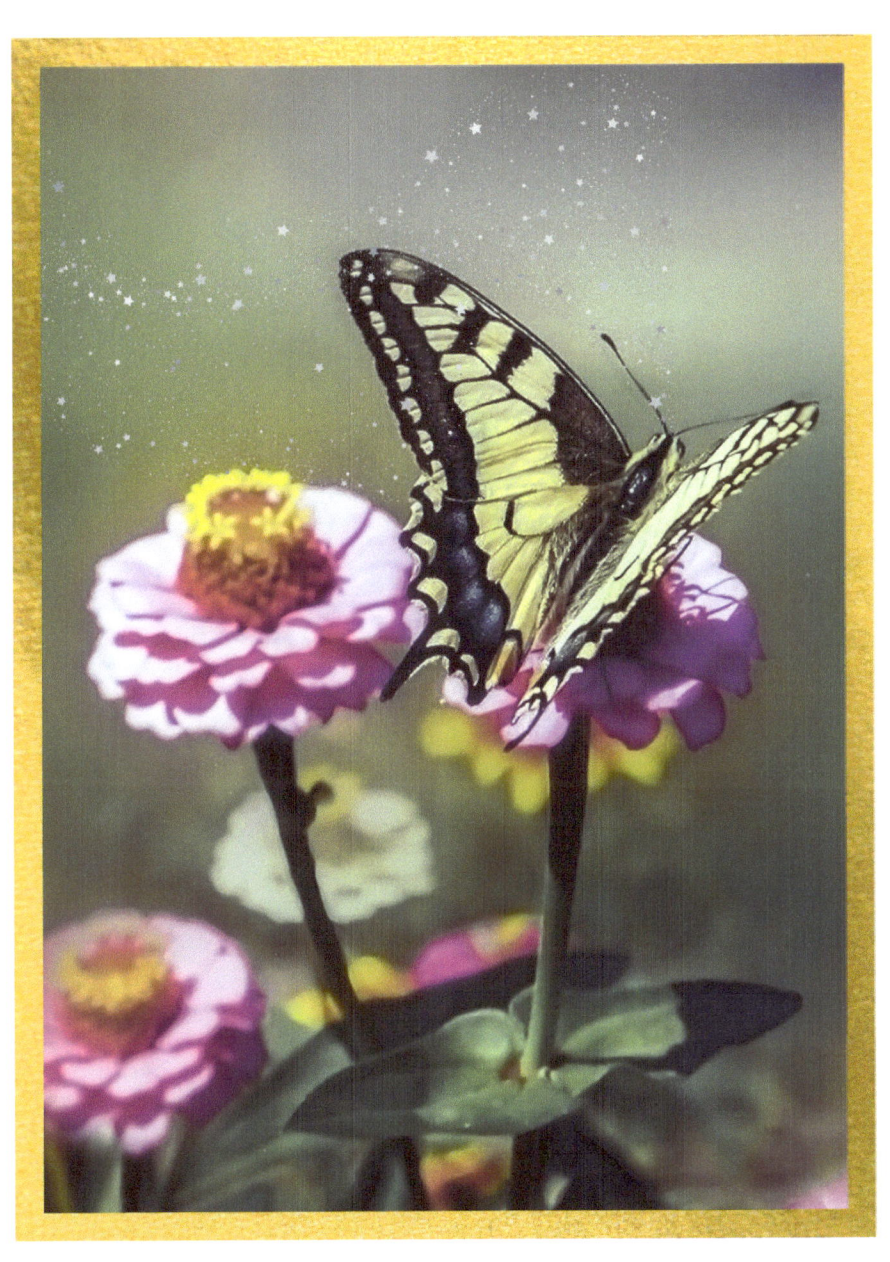

Rest & heal if you need ... ...

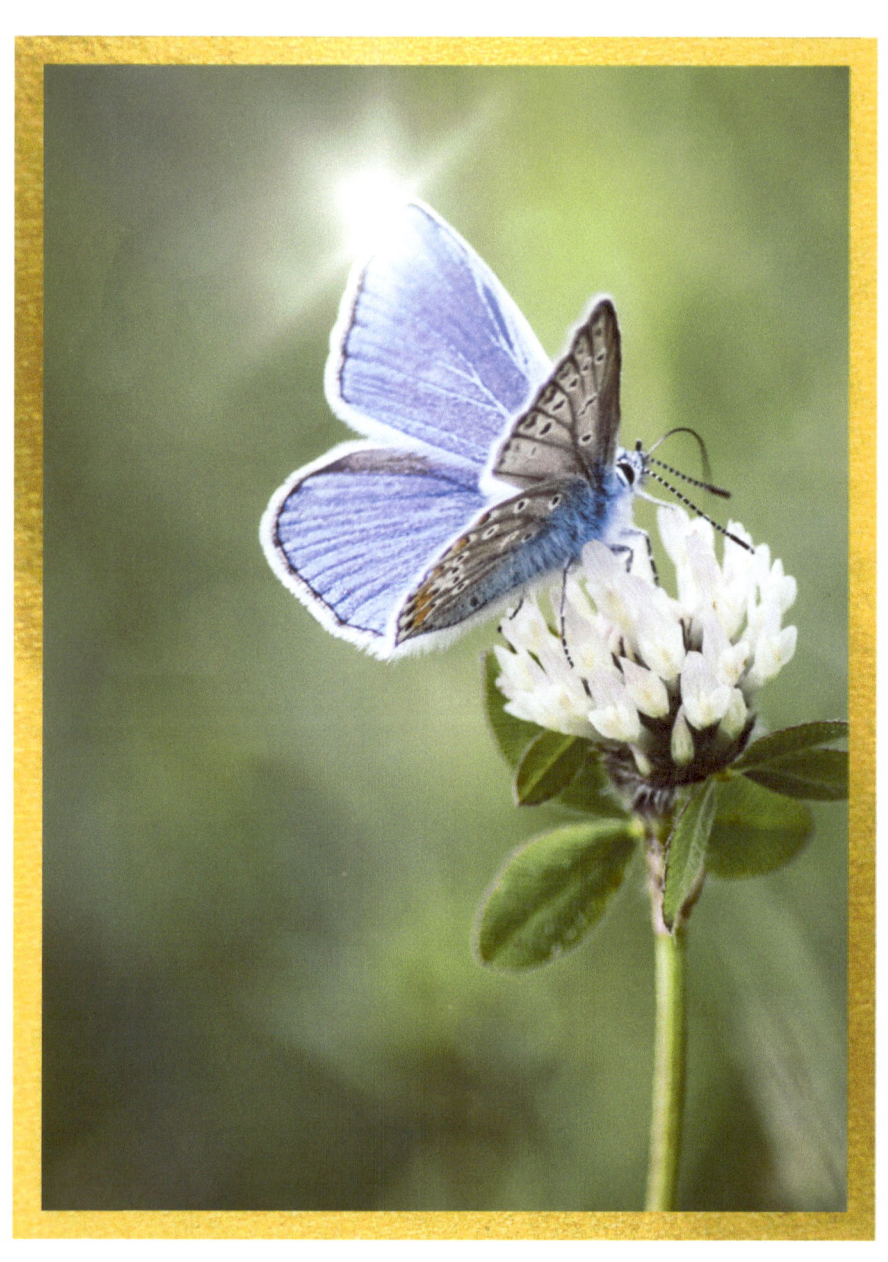

Am I a rare beauty?

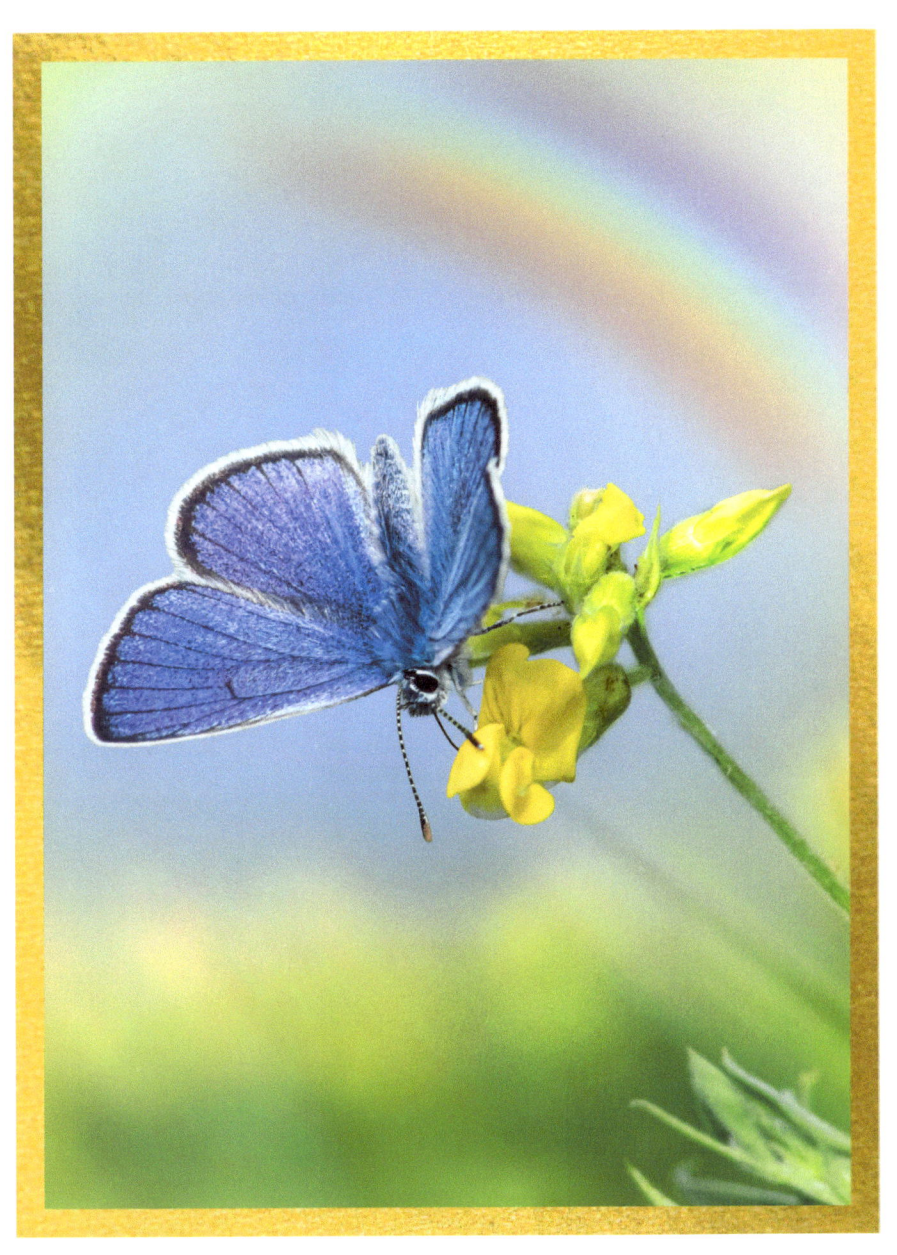

Enjoy the little things

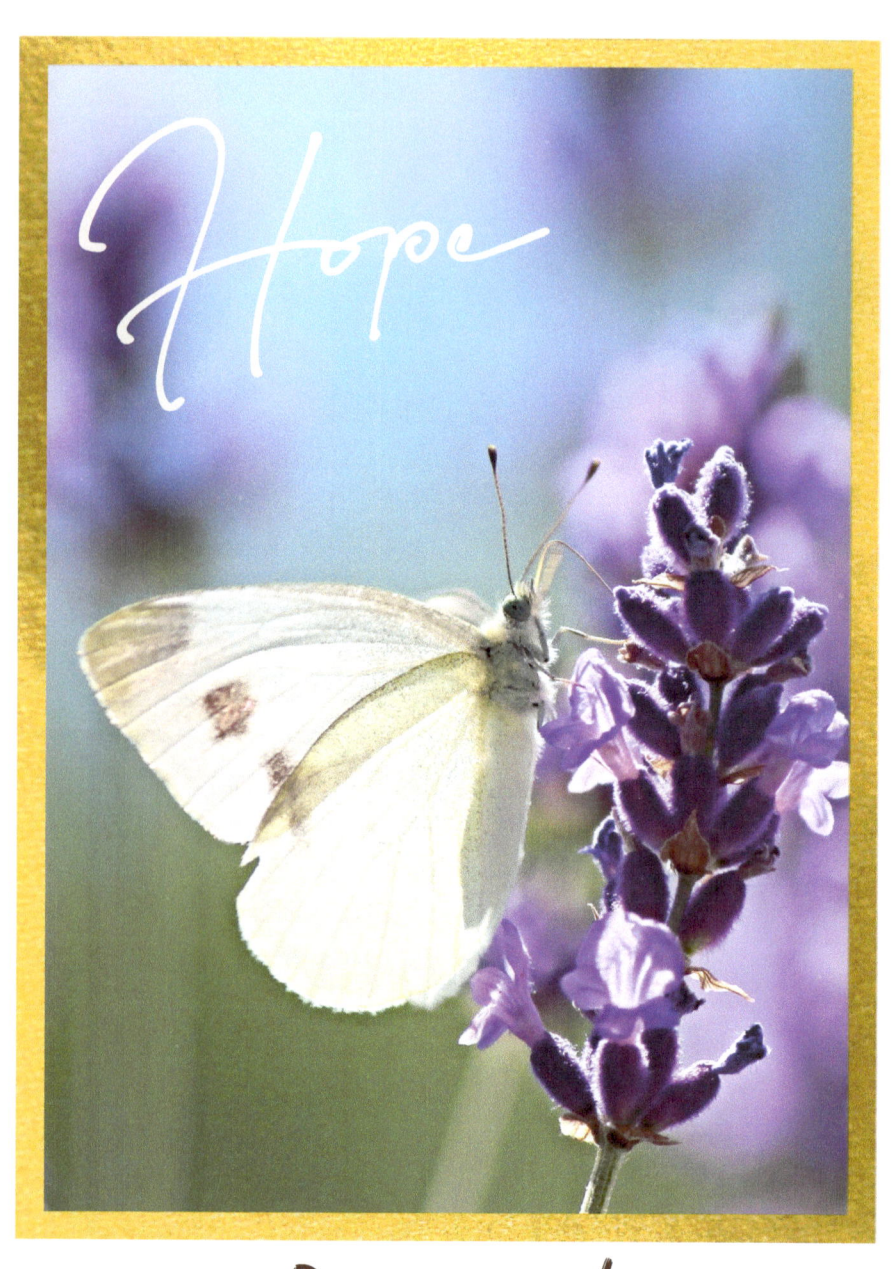

*Hope*

Dear friend,
I wish you a great day!

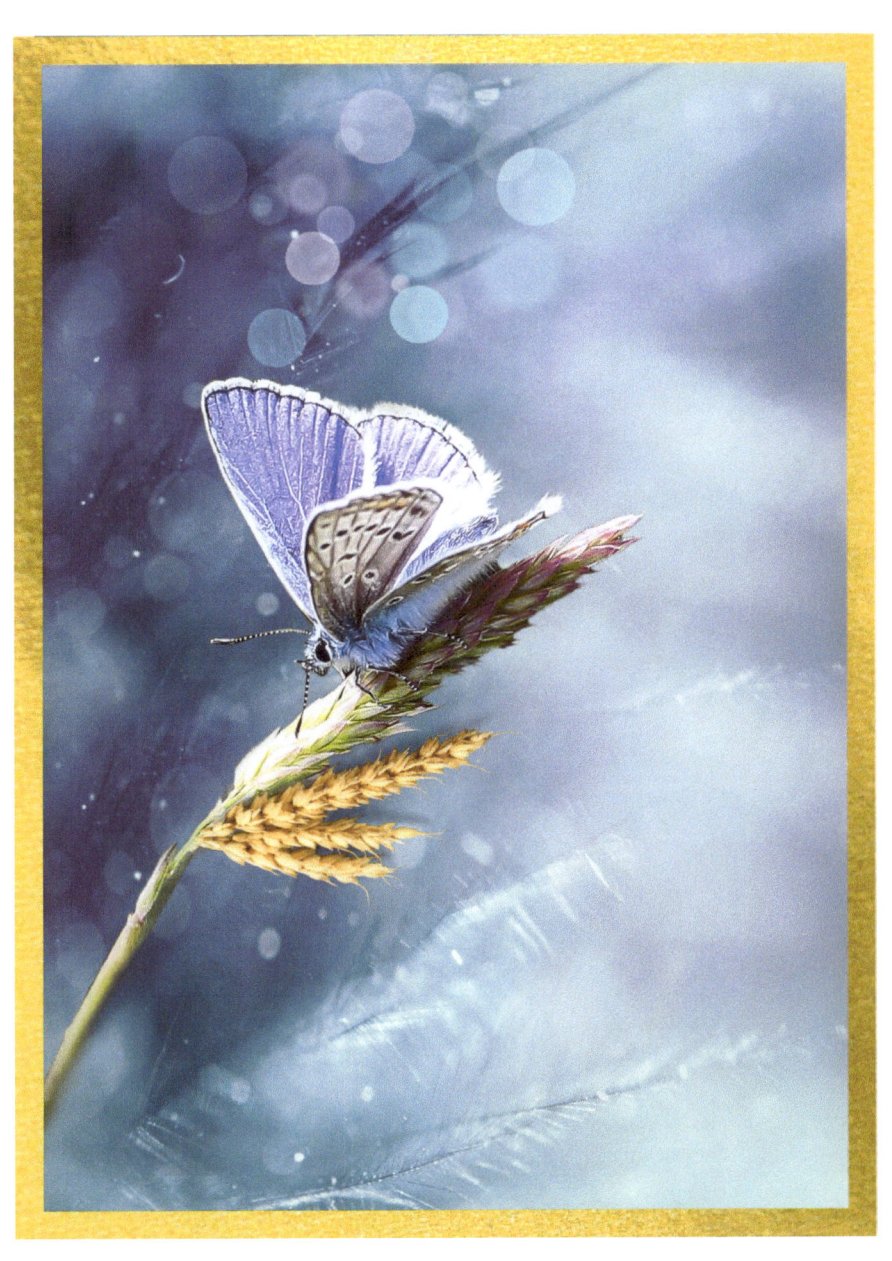

Be kind to yourself

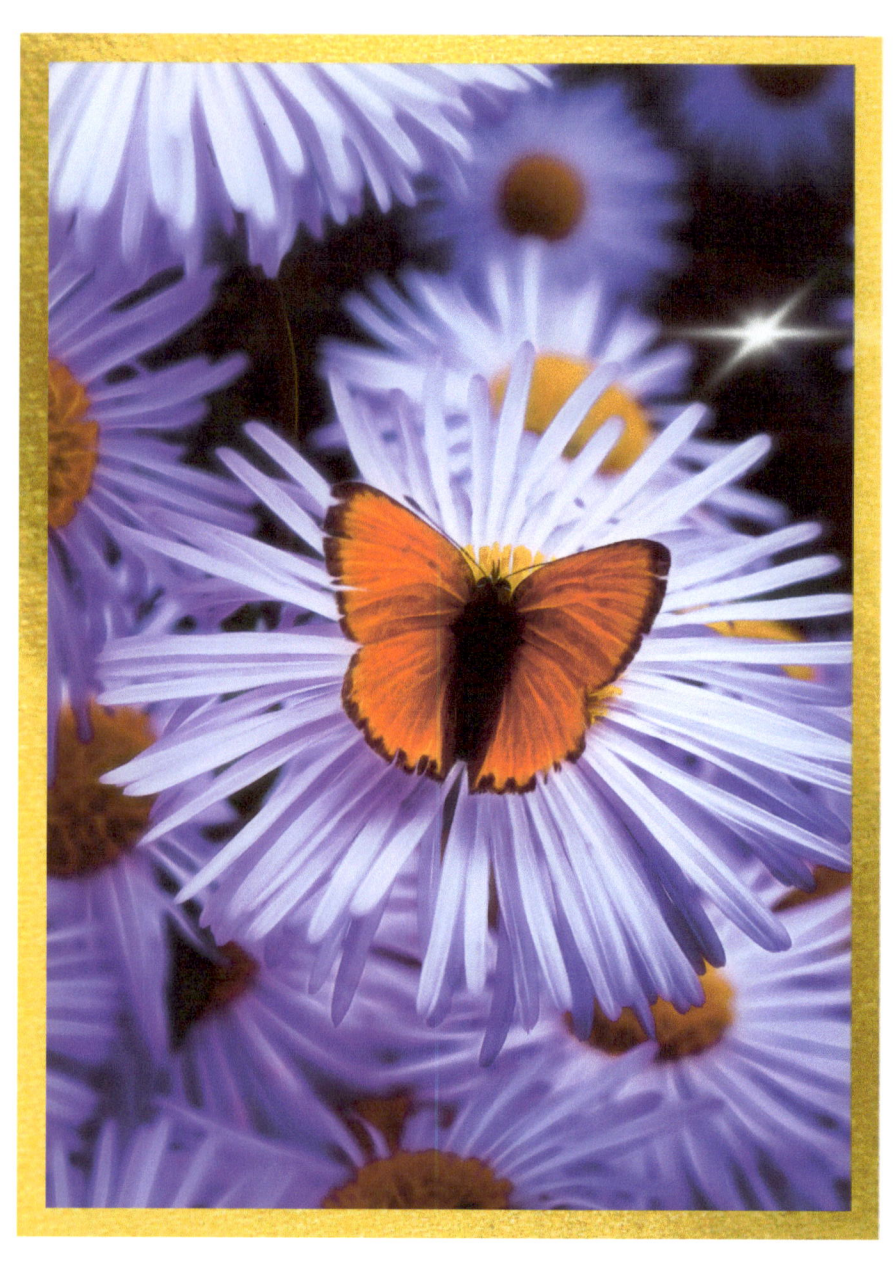

Peace on earth

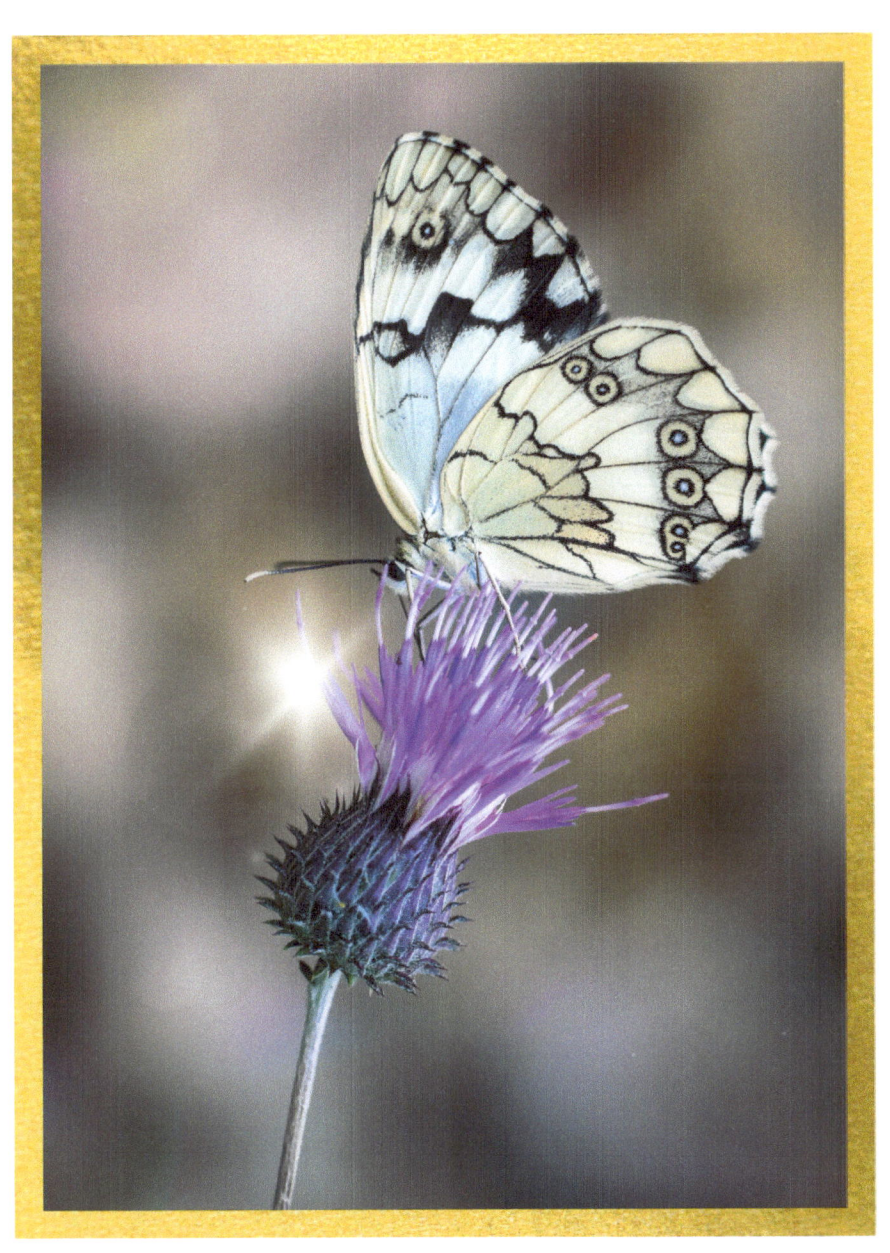

A white beauty!

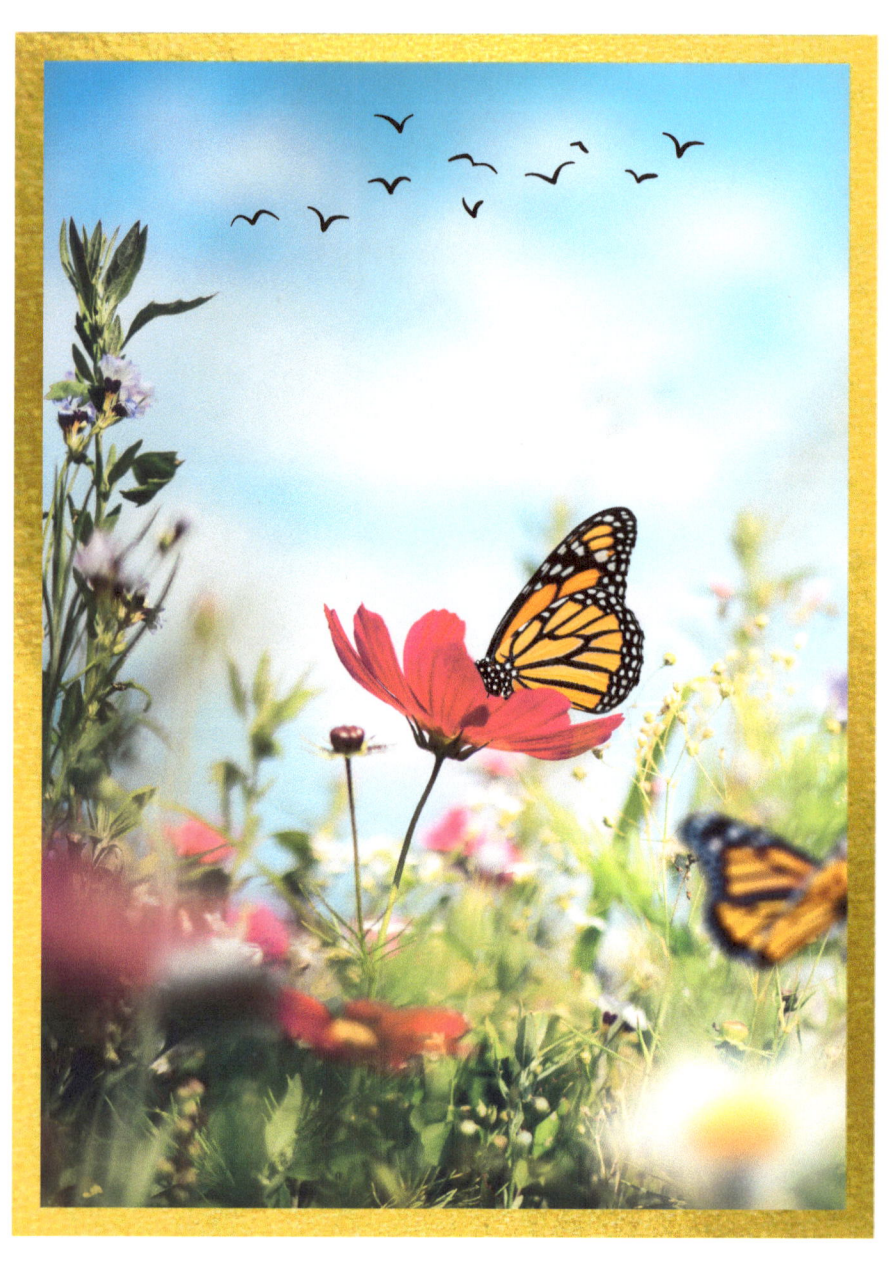

Just relax & smell the roses

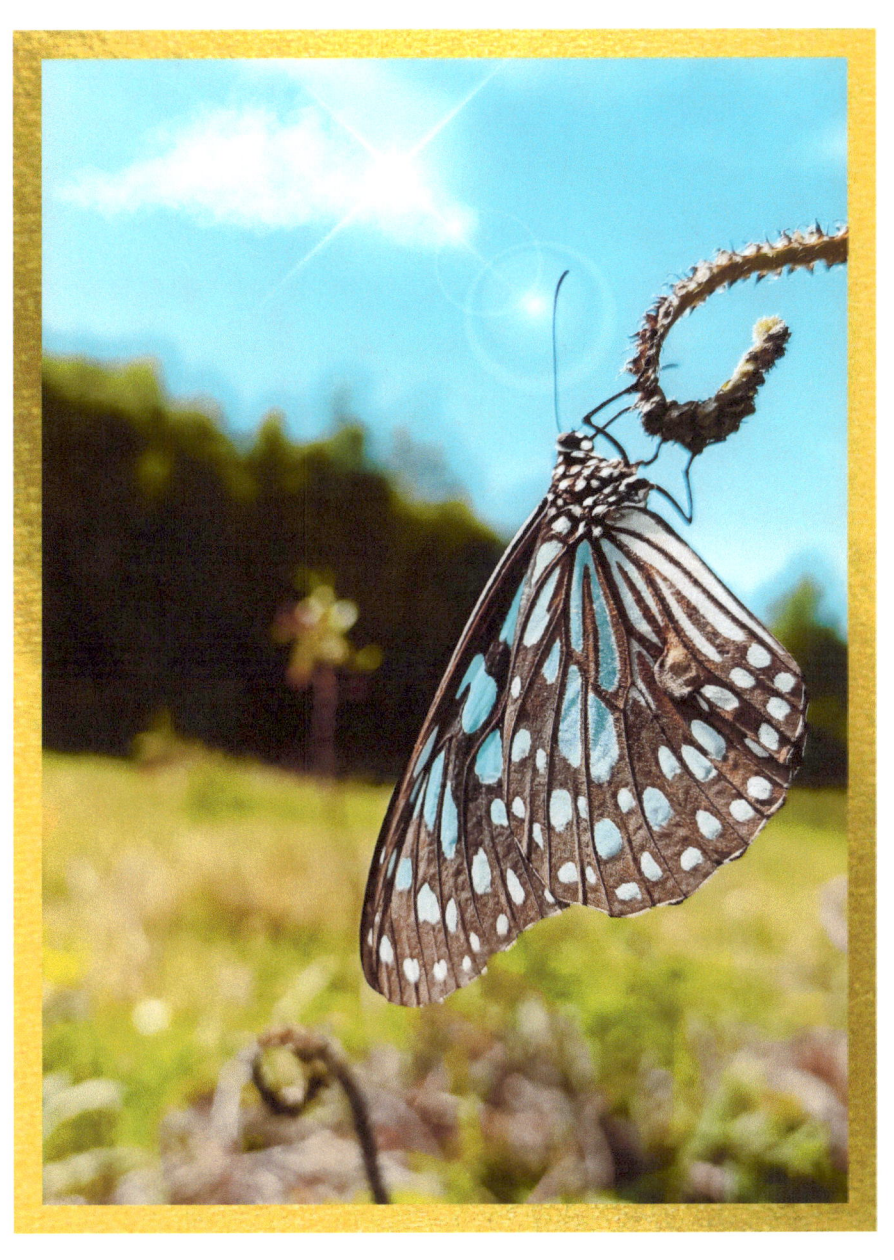

There is always something to strive for

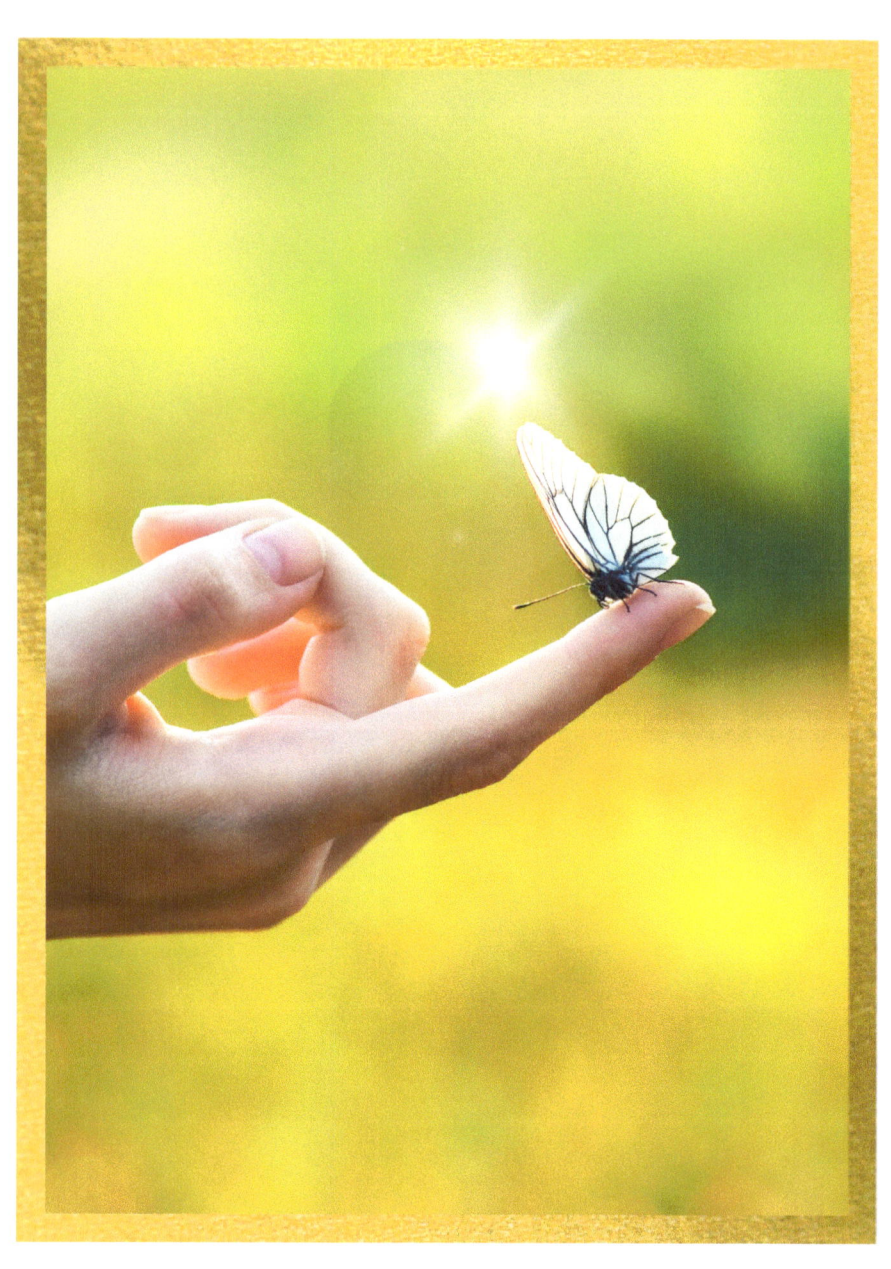

Hi! I love you.

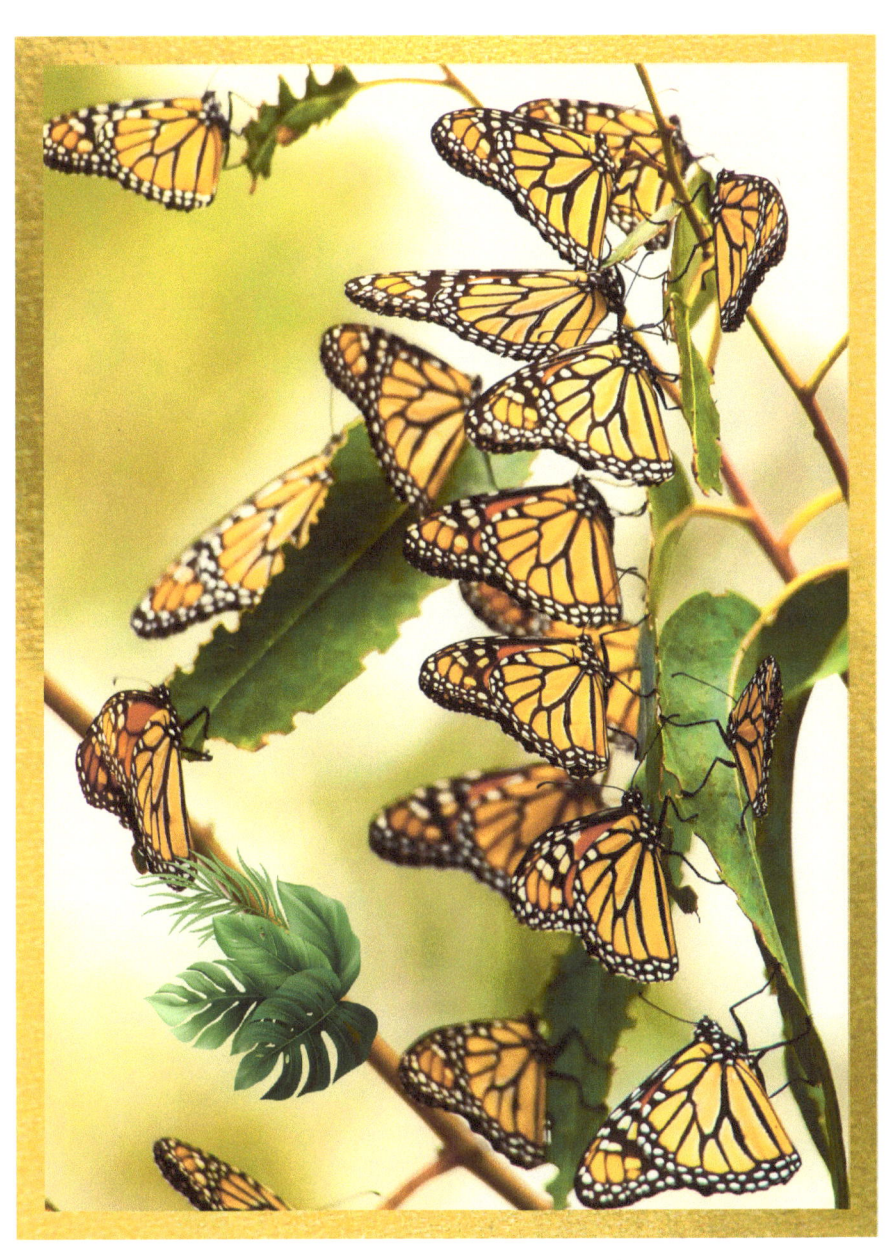

That's what friends are for!

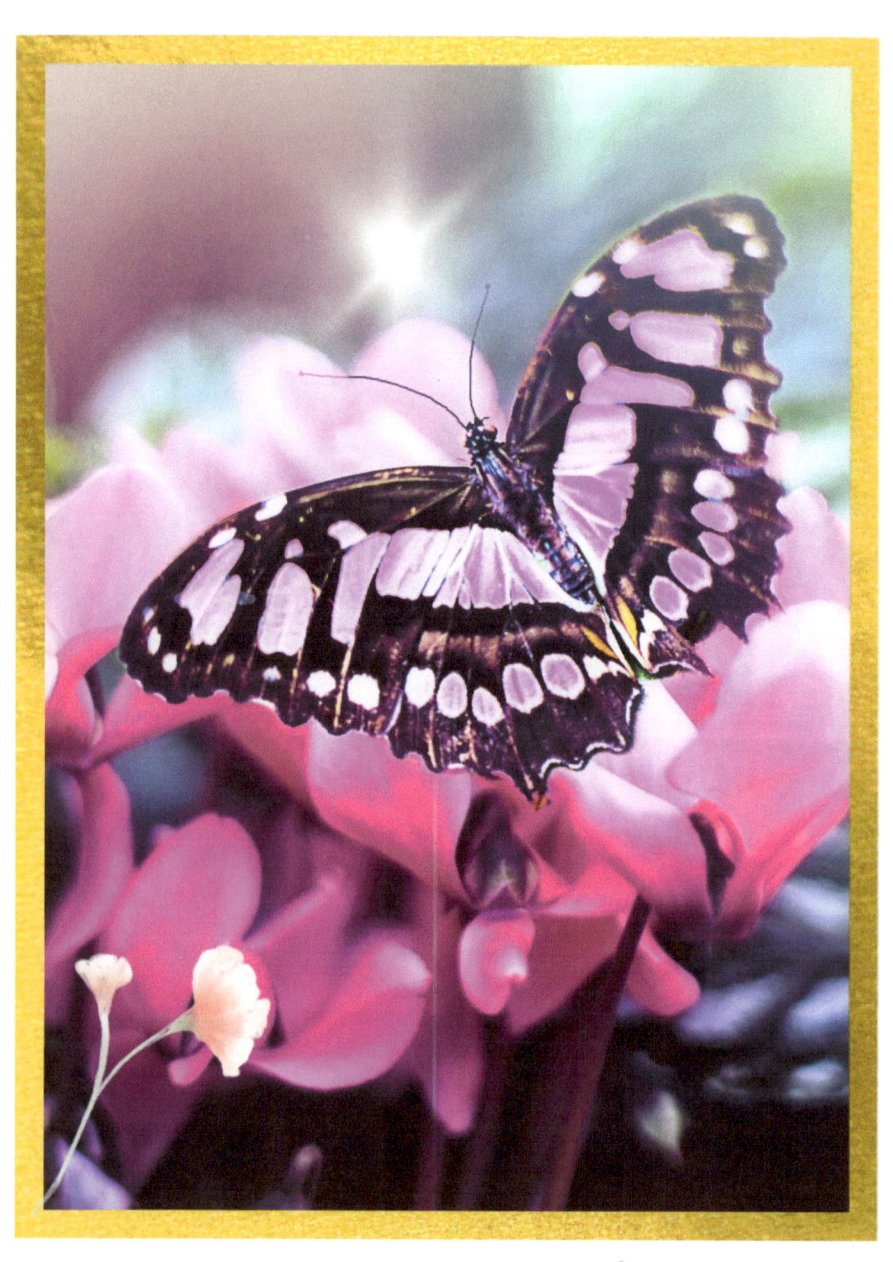

Dear Friend,
I wish you a good day!

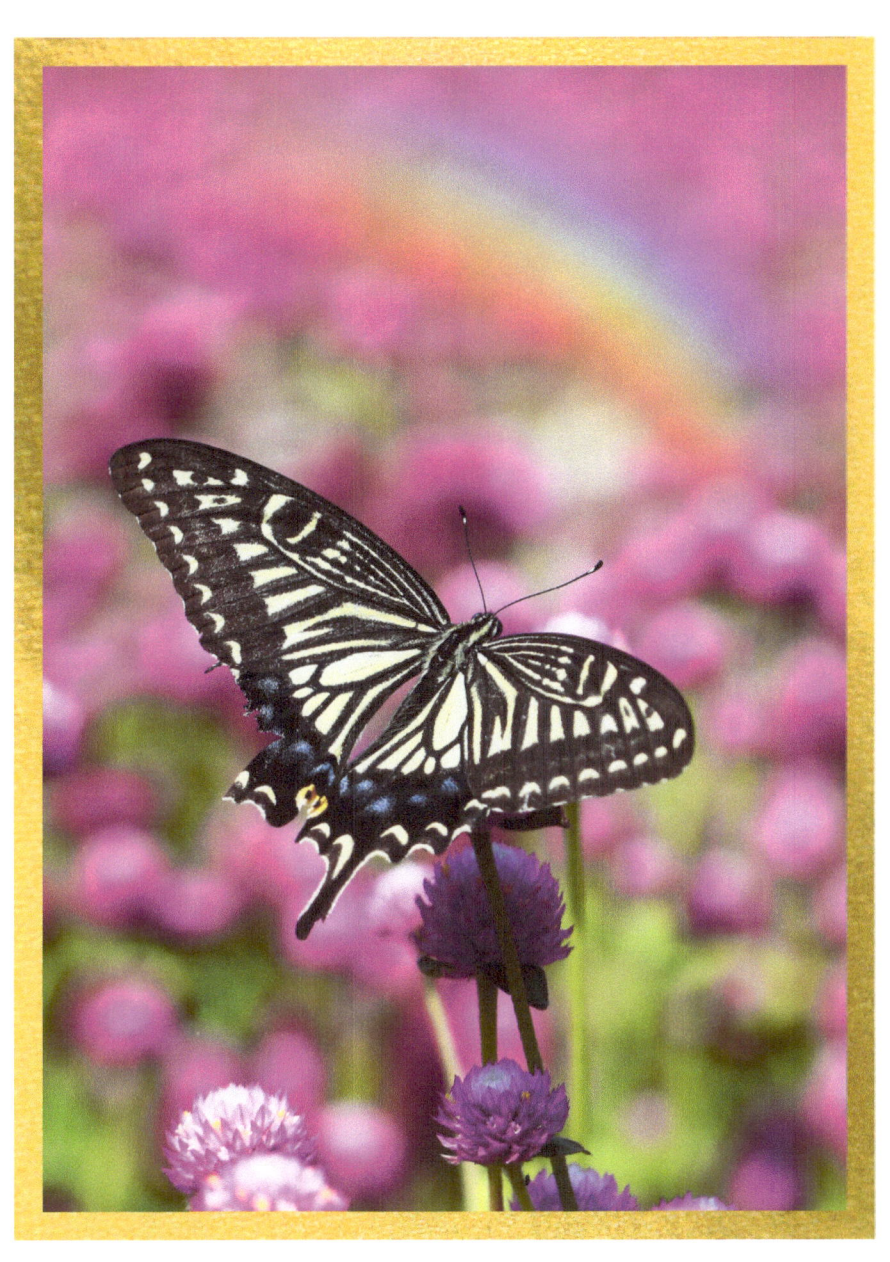

Elegance in the nature

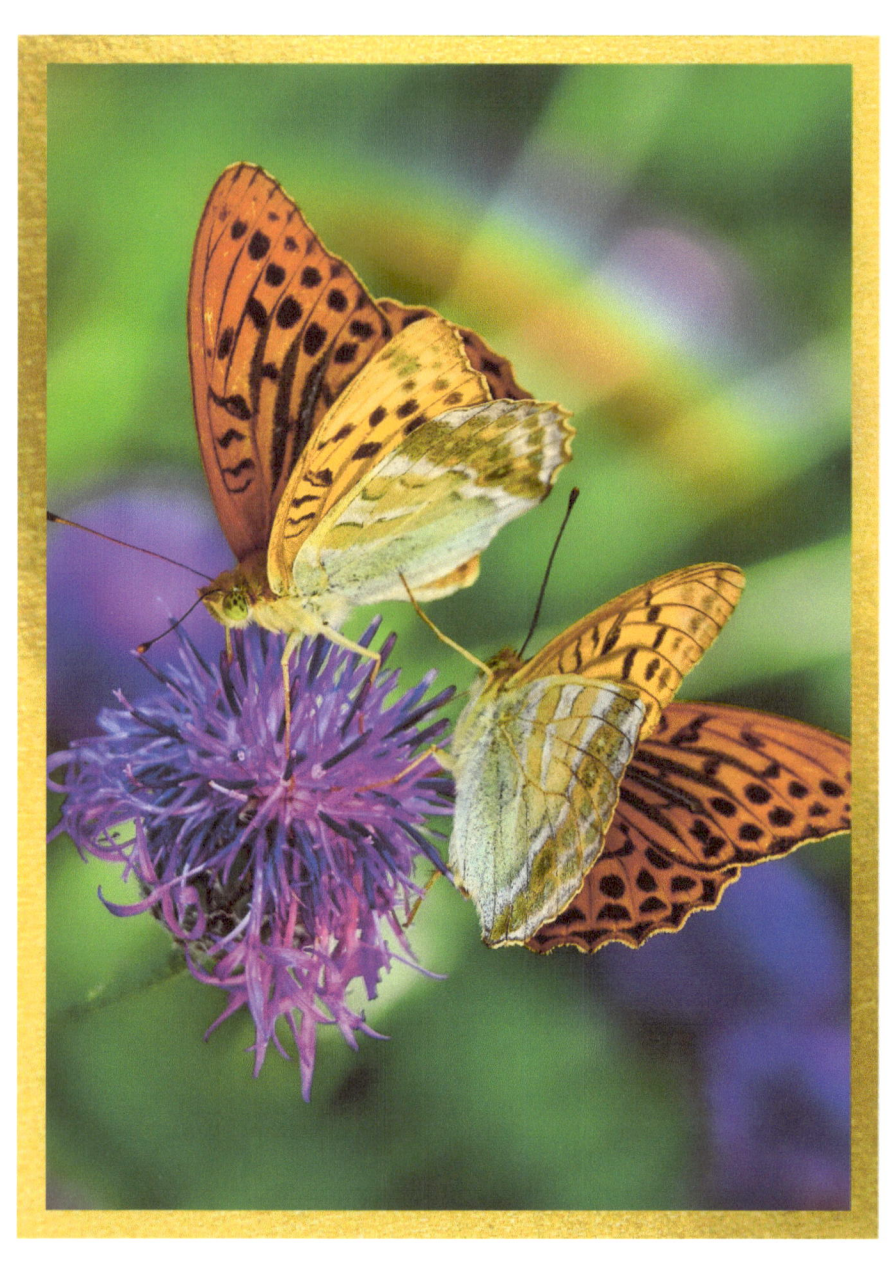

*Life is beautiful!*

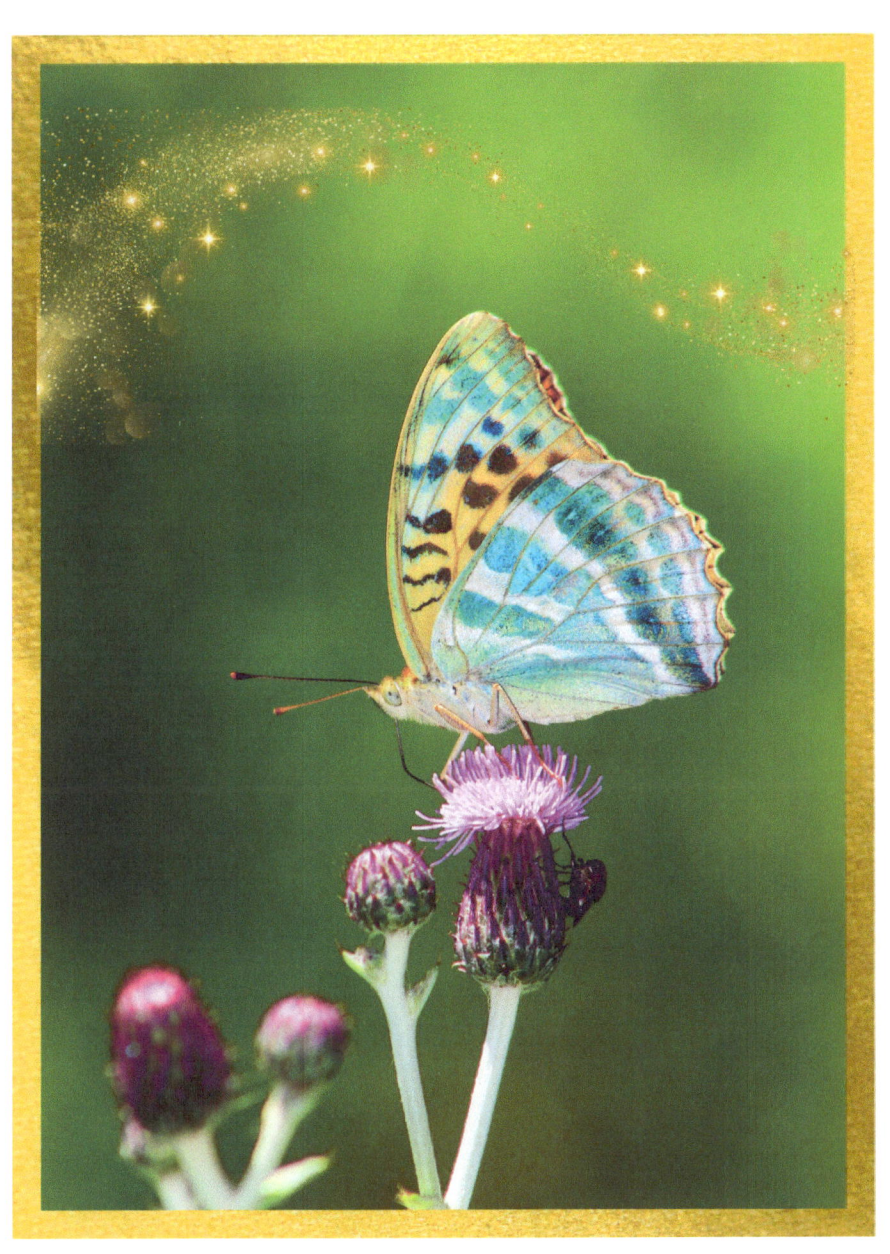

This is the best day

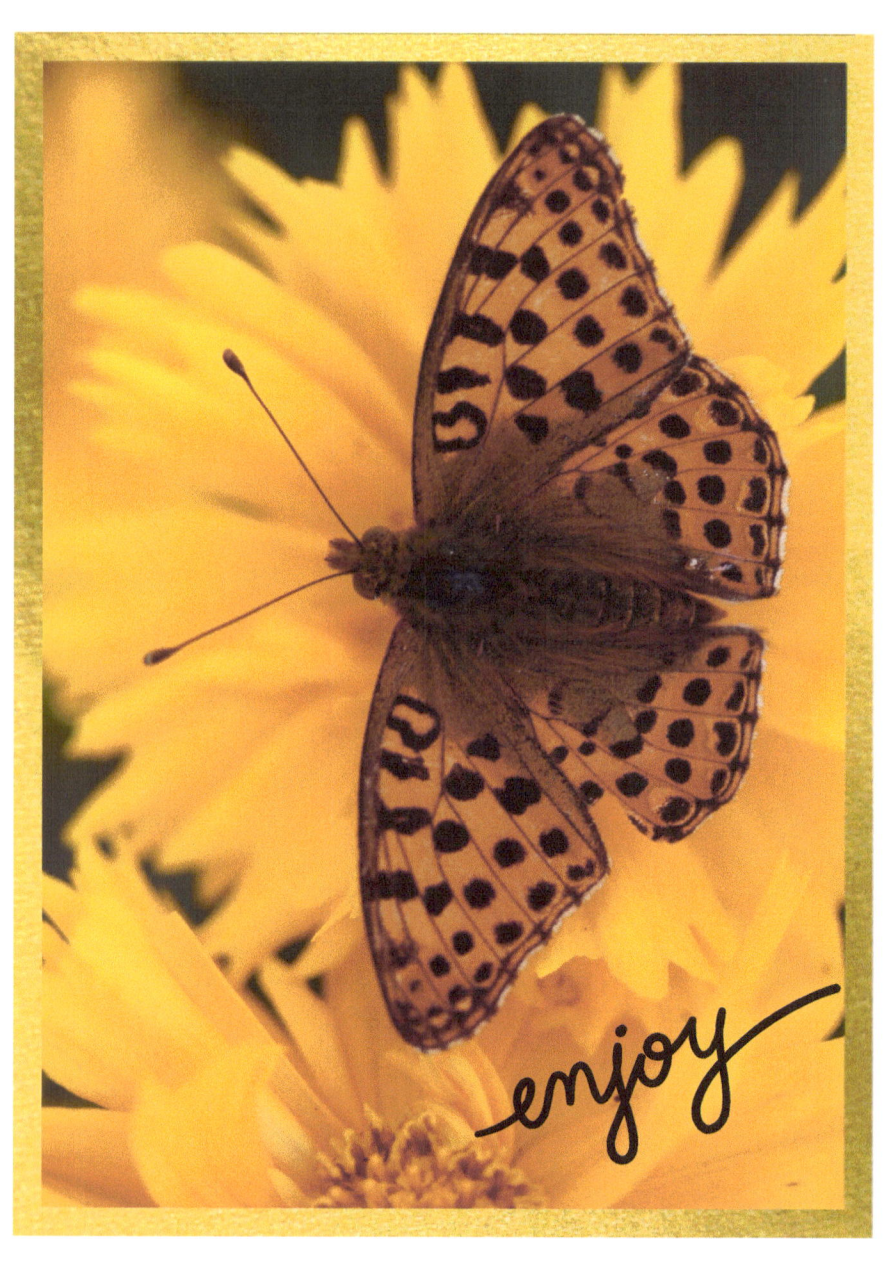

*enjoy*

Be completely still & enjoy this moment

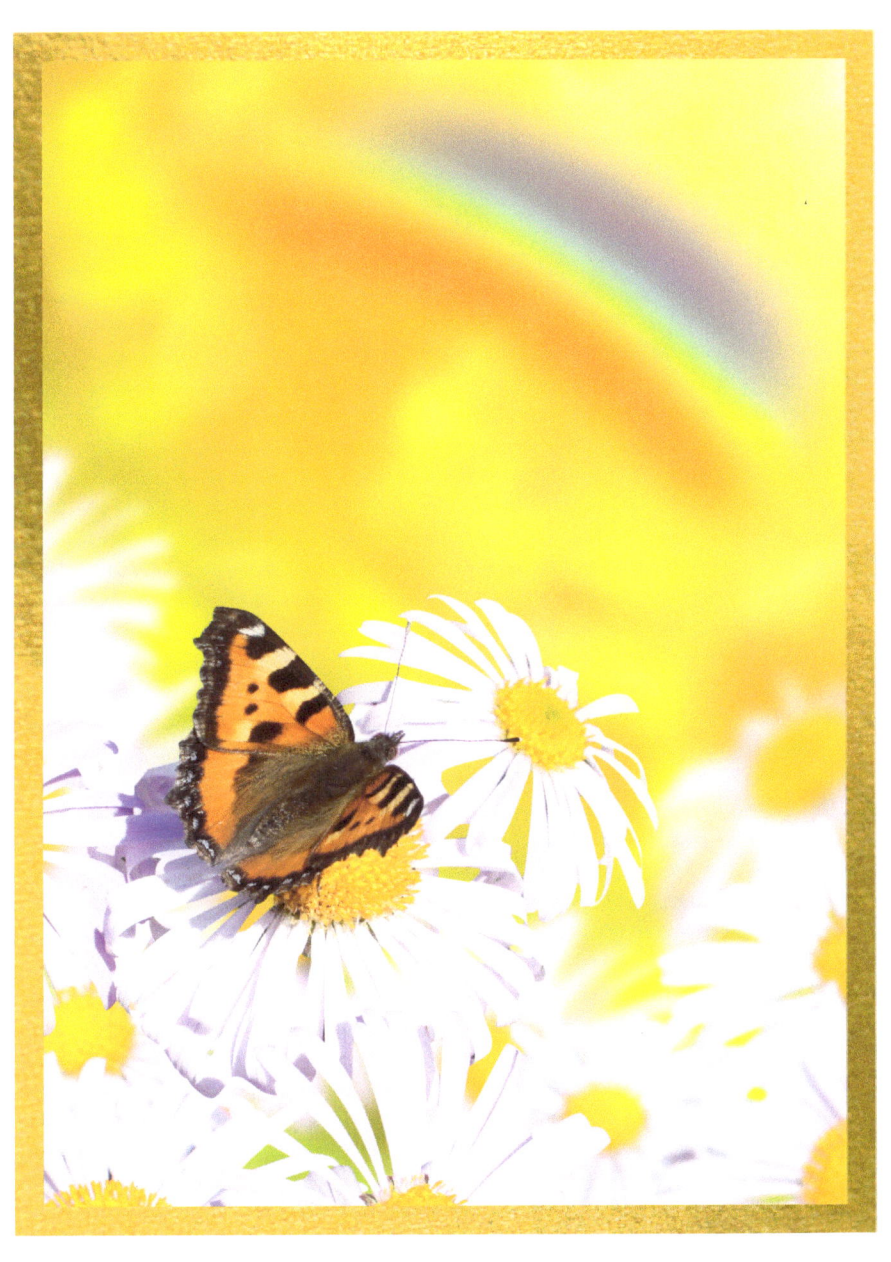

I love the golden morning rays!

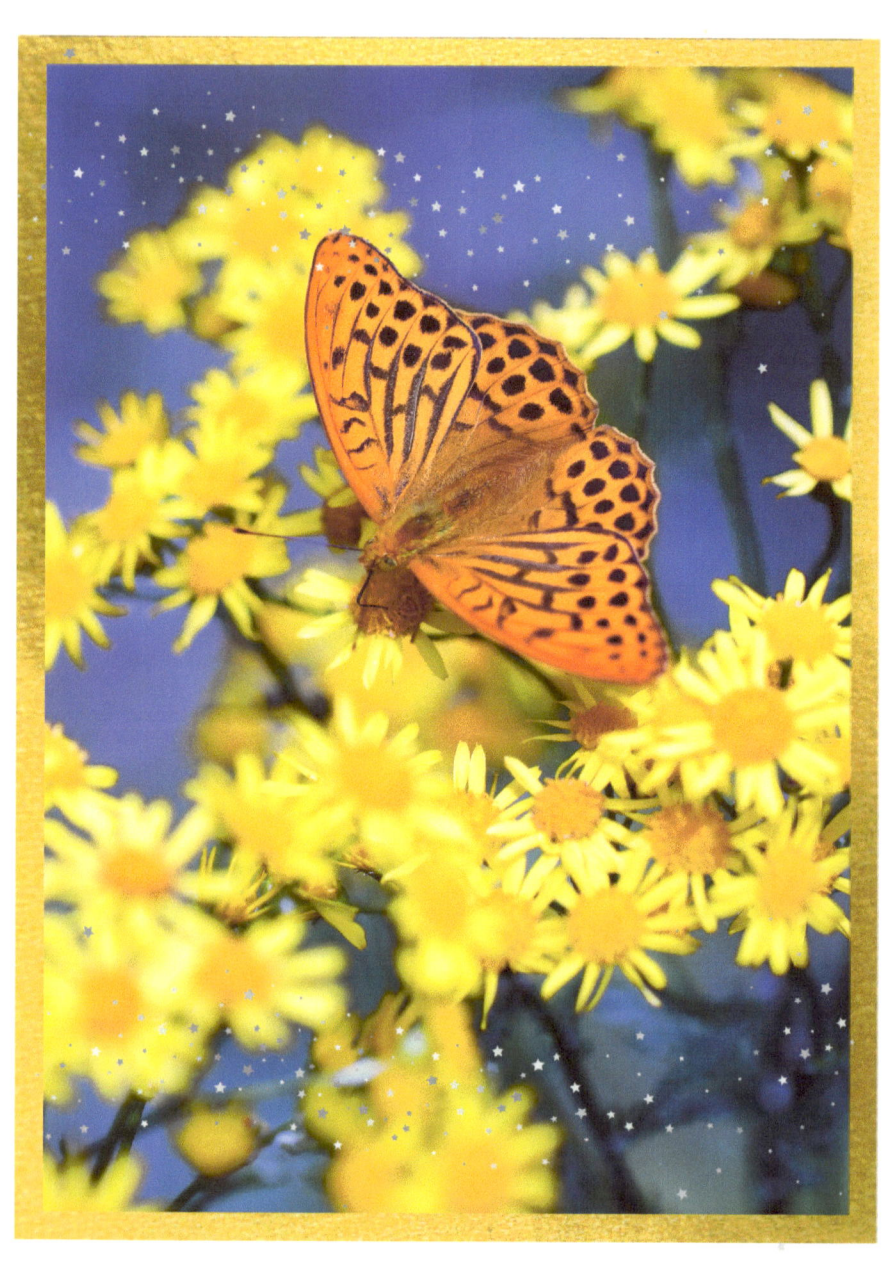

You are surrounded by grace

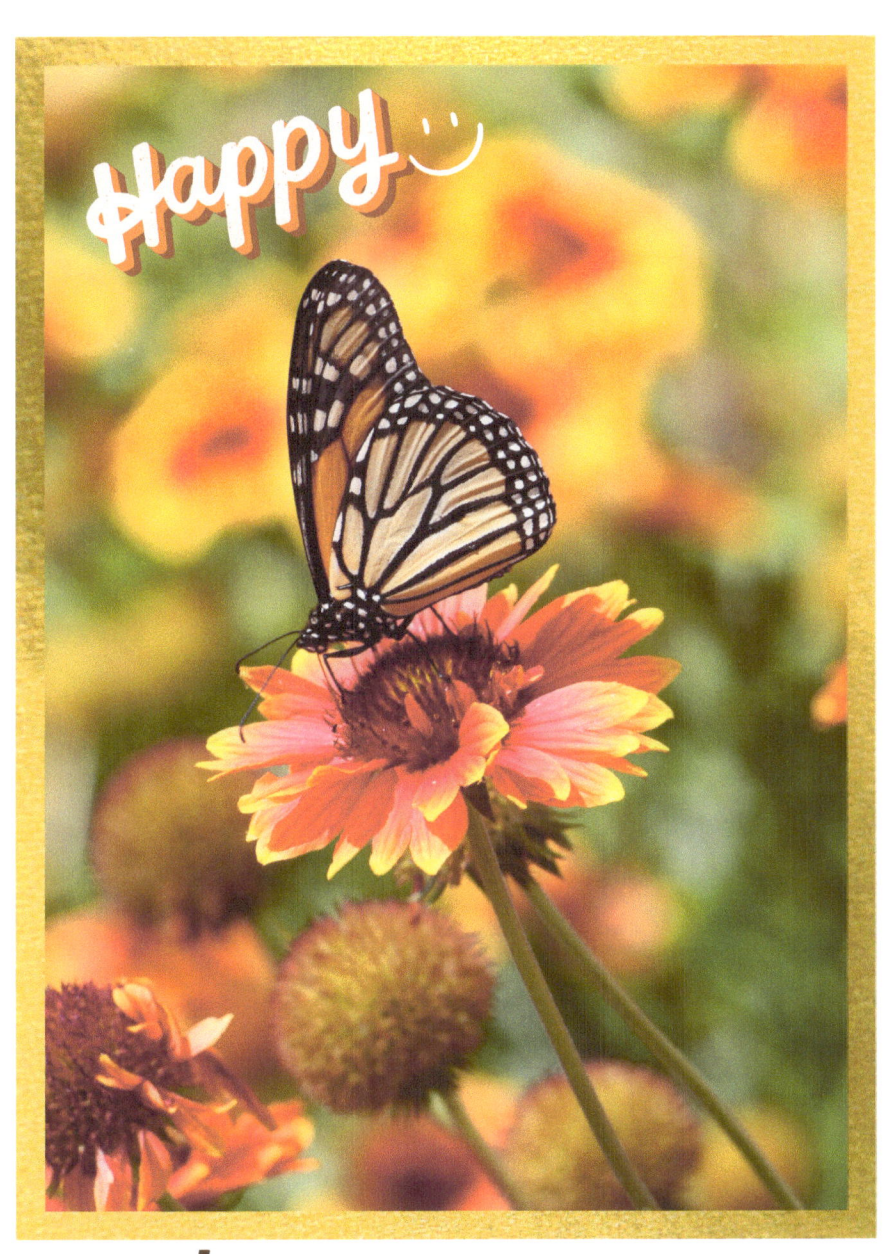

Happy :)

I' m happy only when
I m in nature

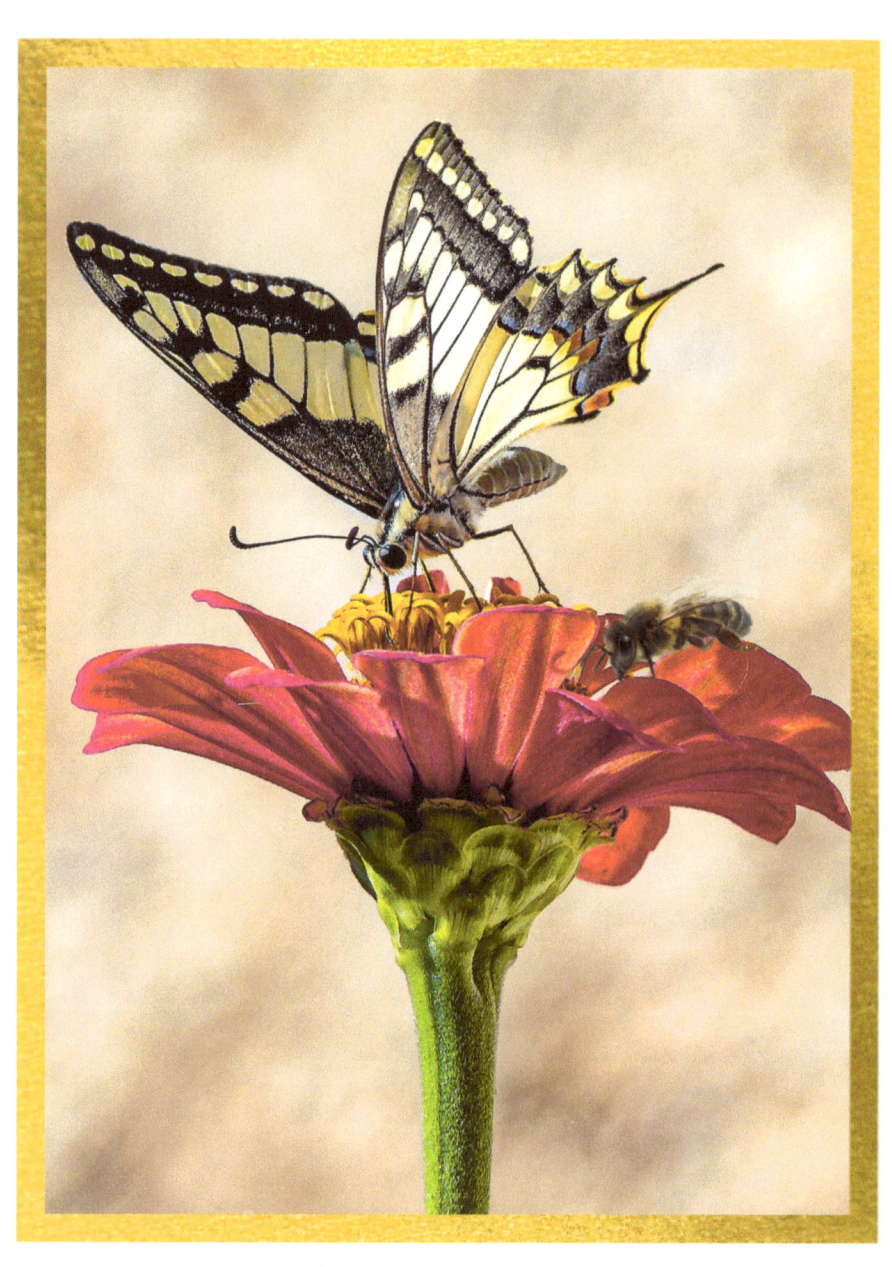

Chill & smell the flower

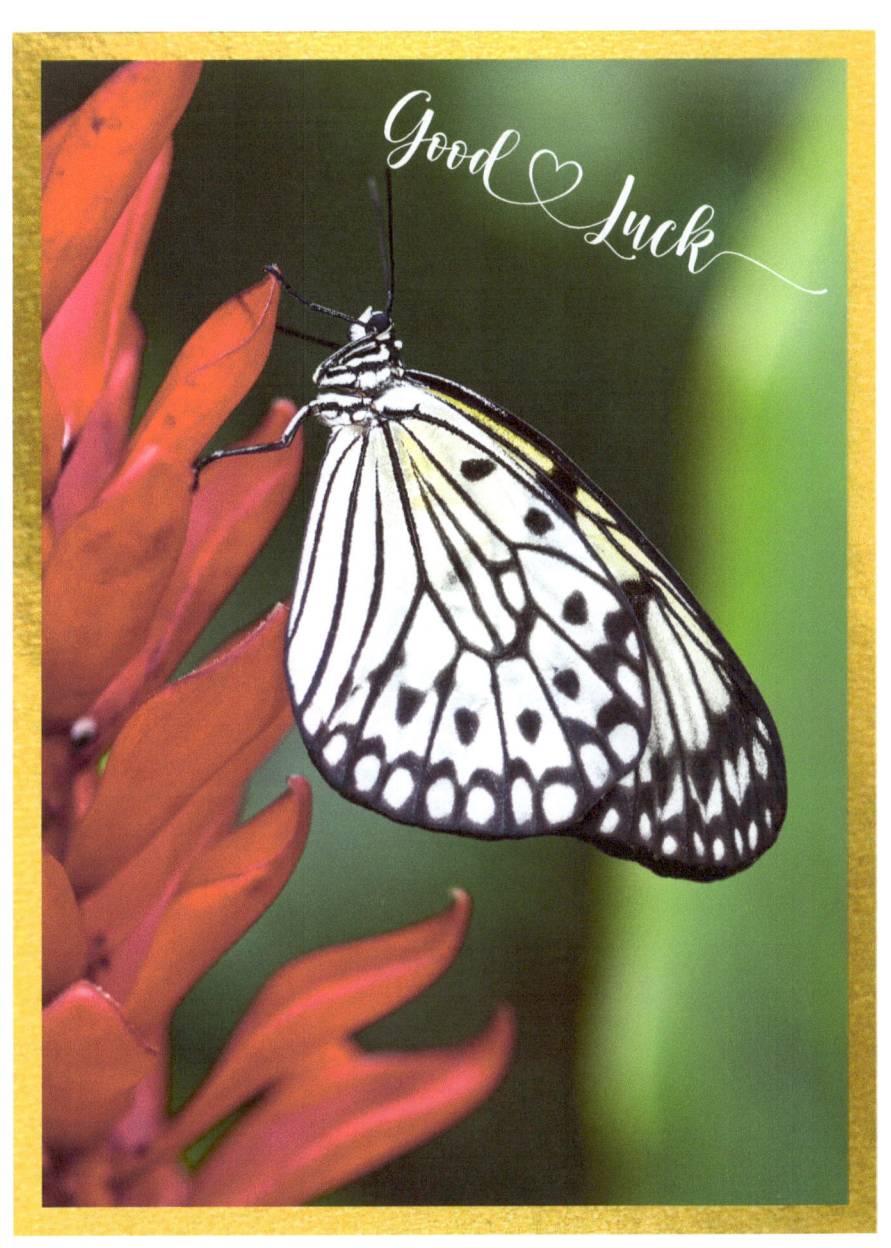

Good ♡ Luck

An awesome day to you!

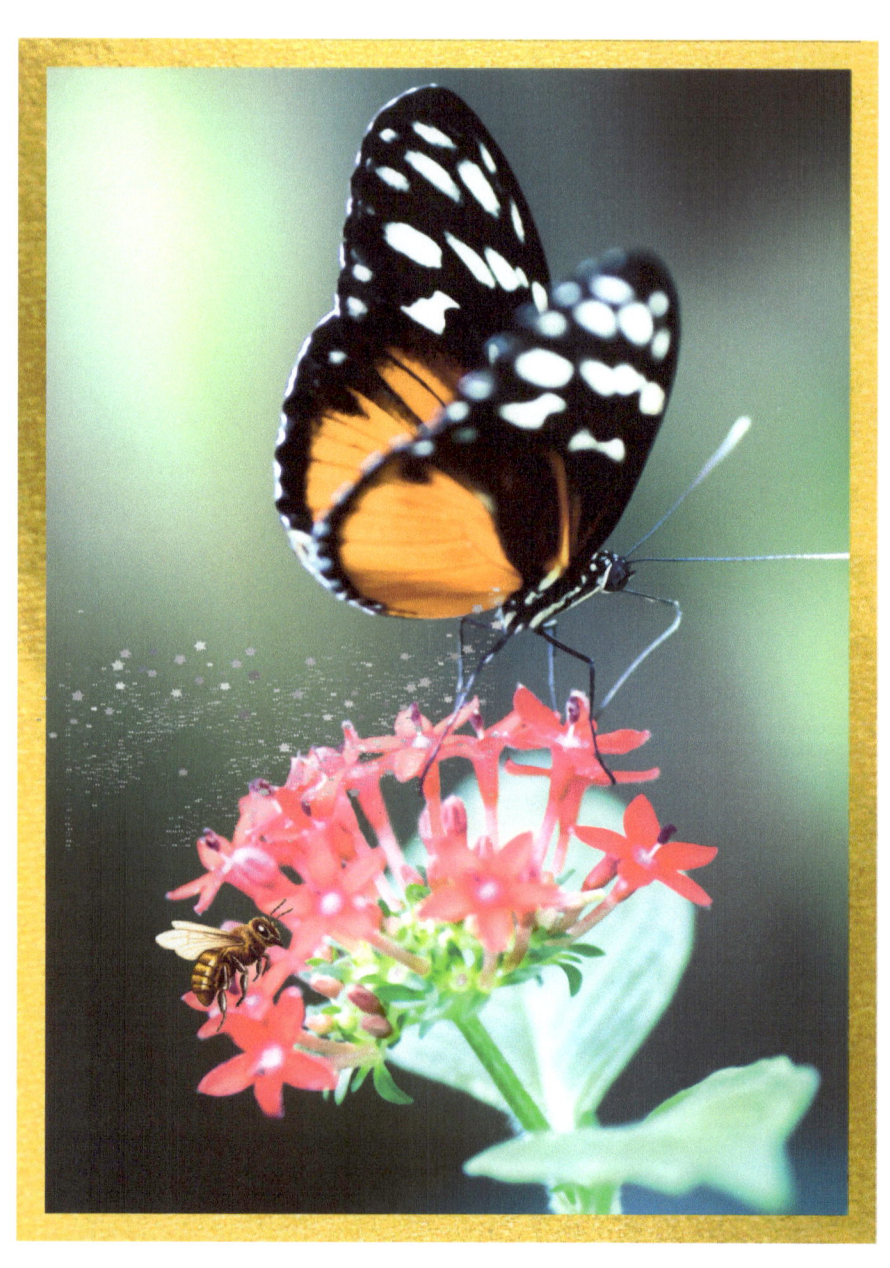

*Everyone has his own place in life*

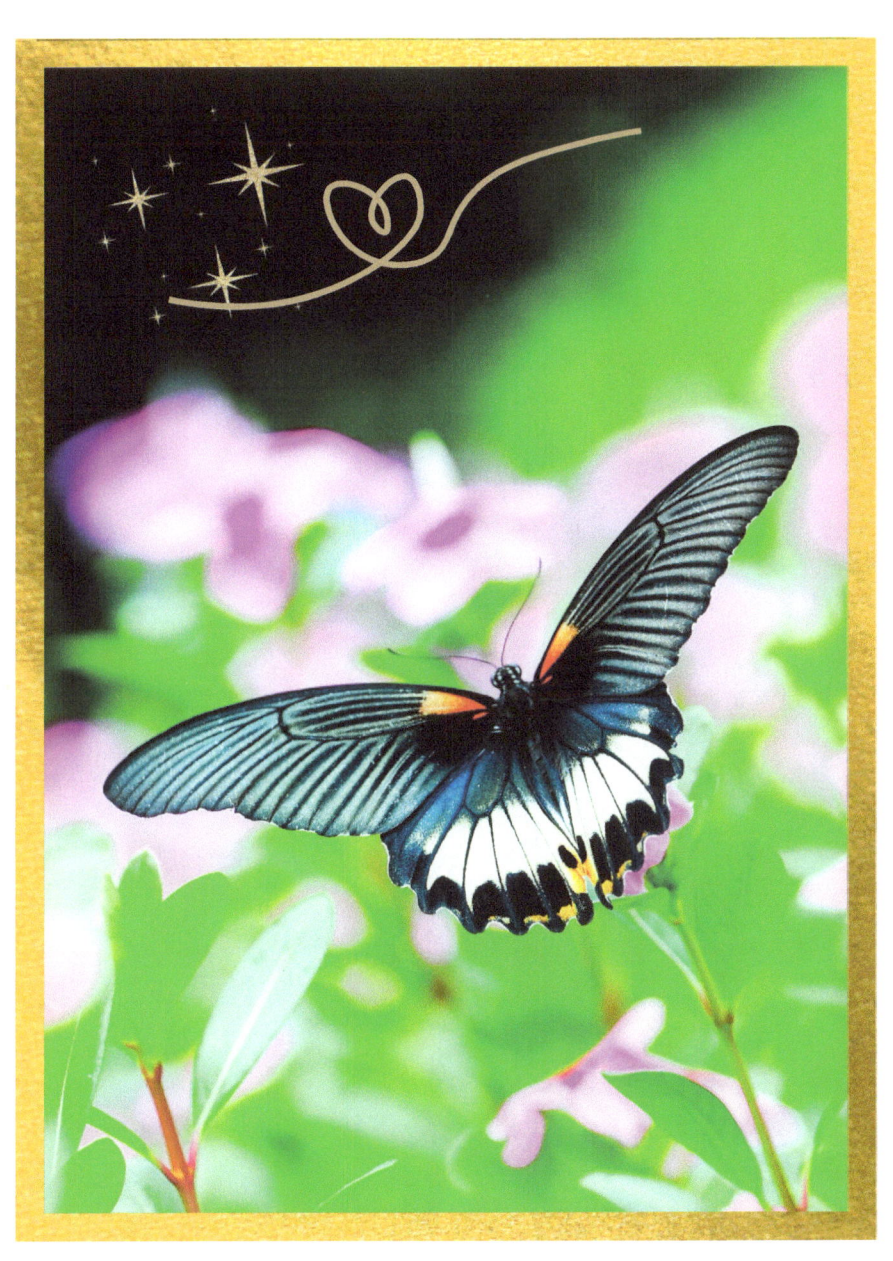

May you be well & happy!

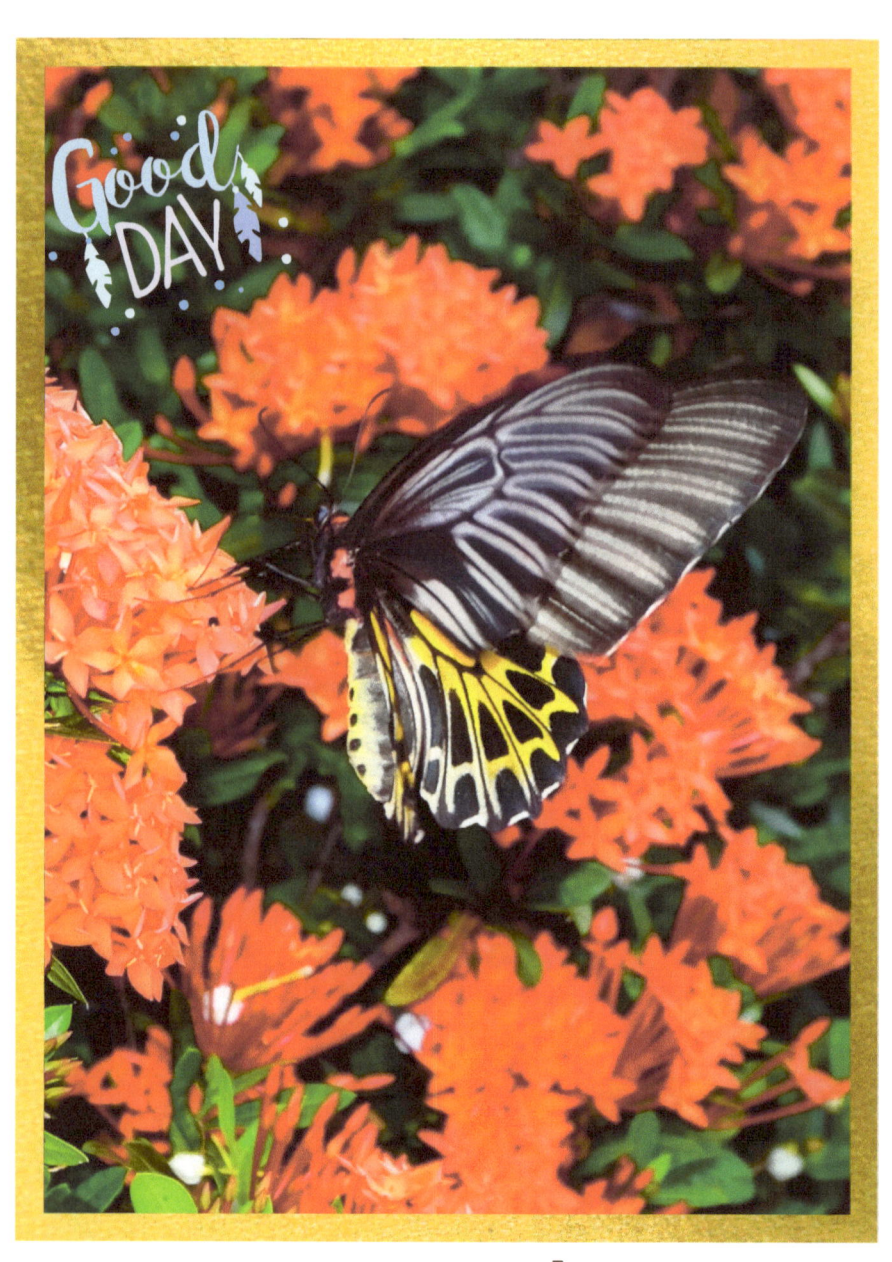

Nature has it's own
perfect combination

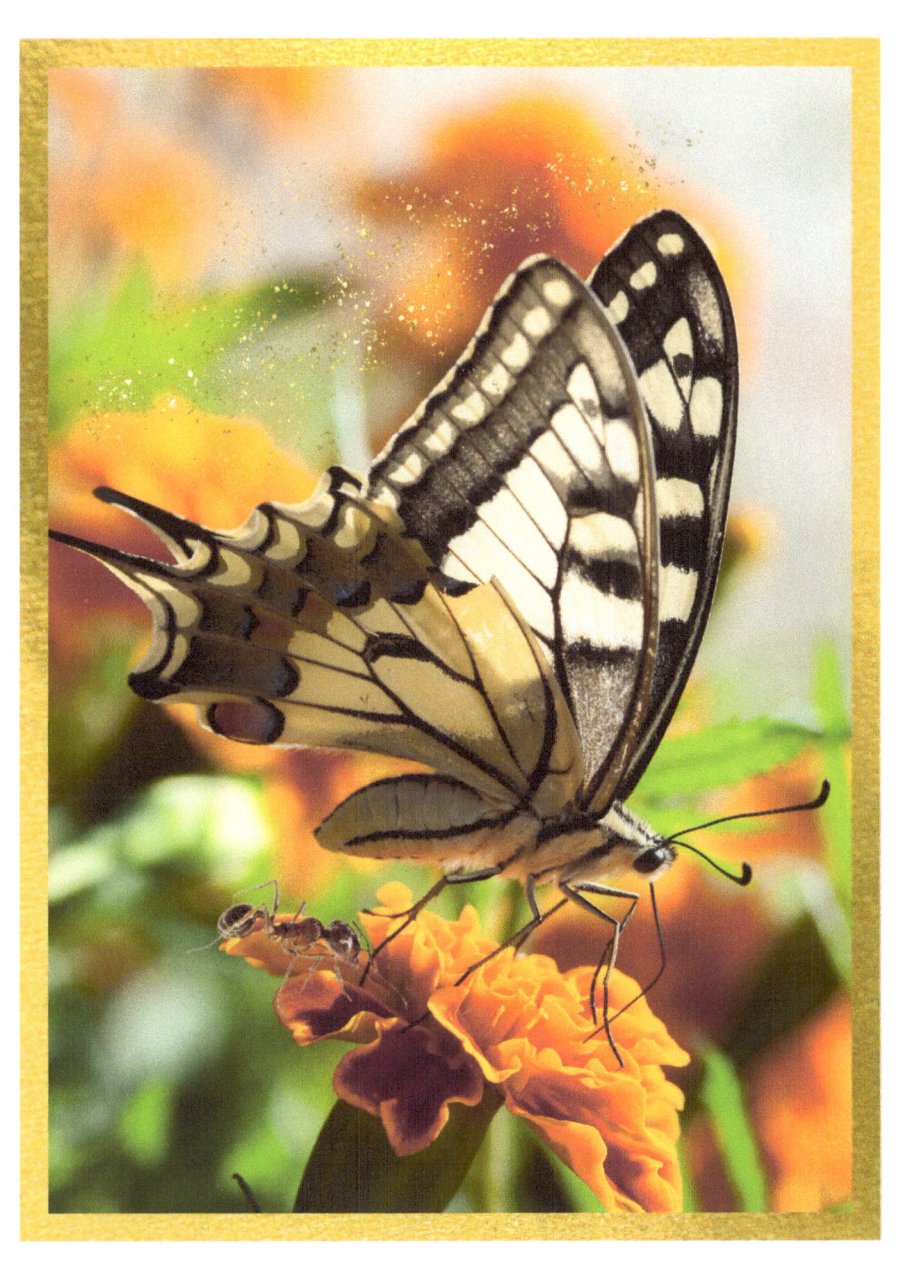

I love to share this beauty with you

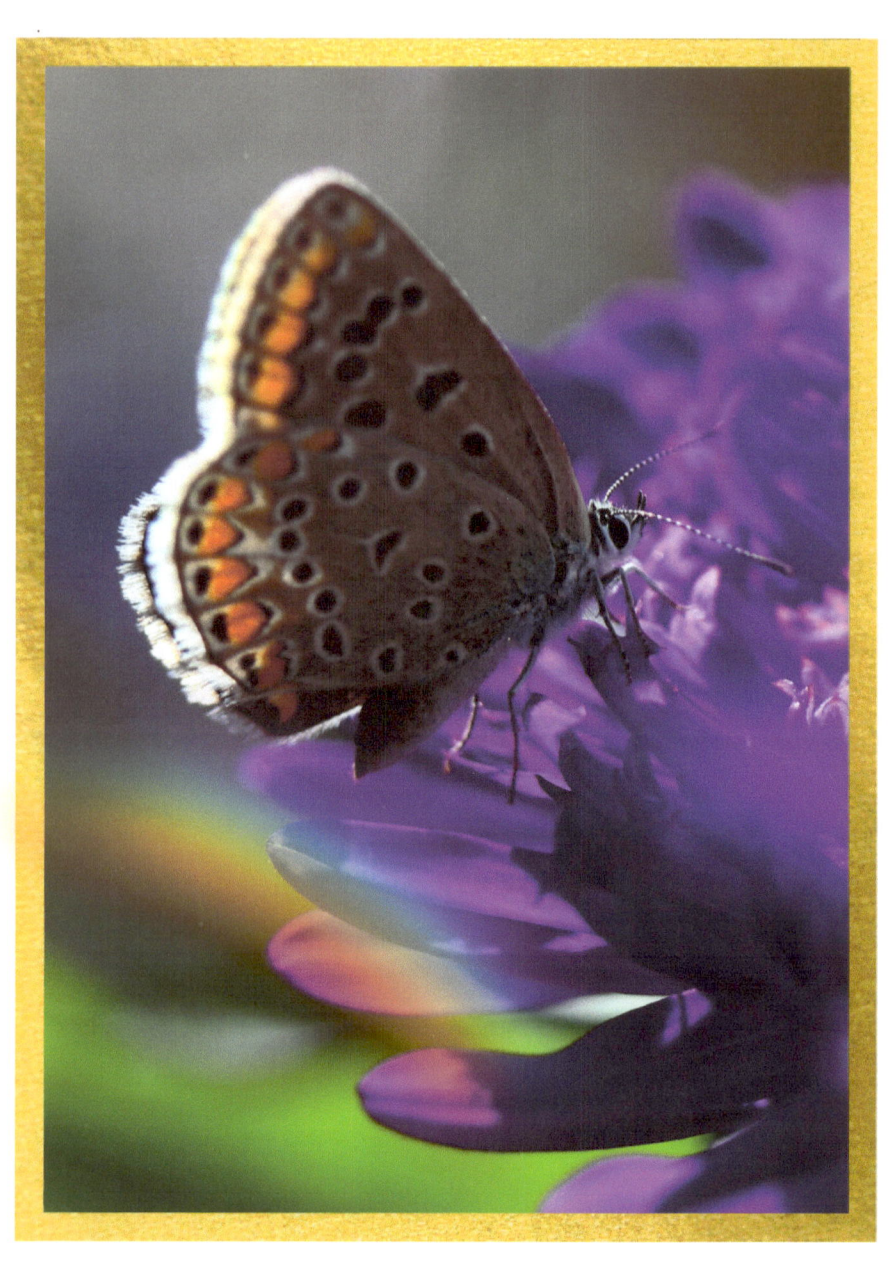

I love this flower. Do you?

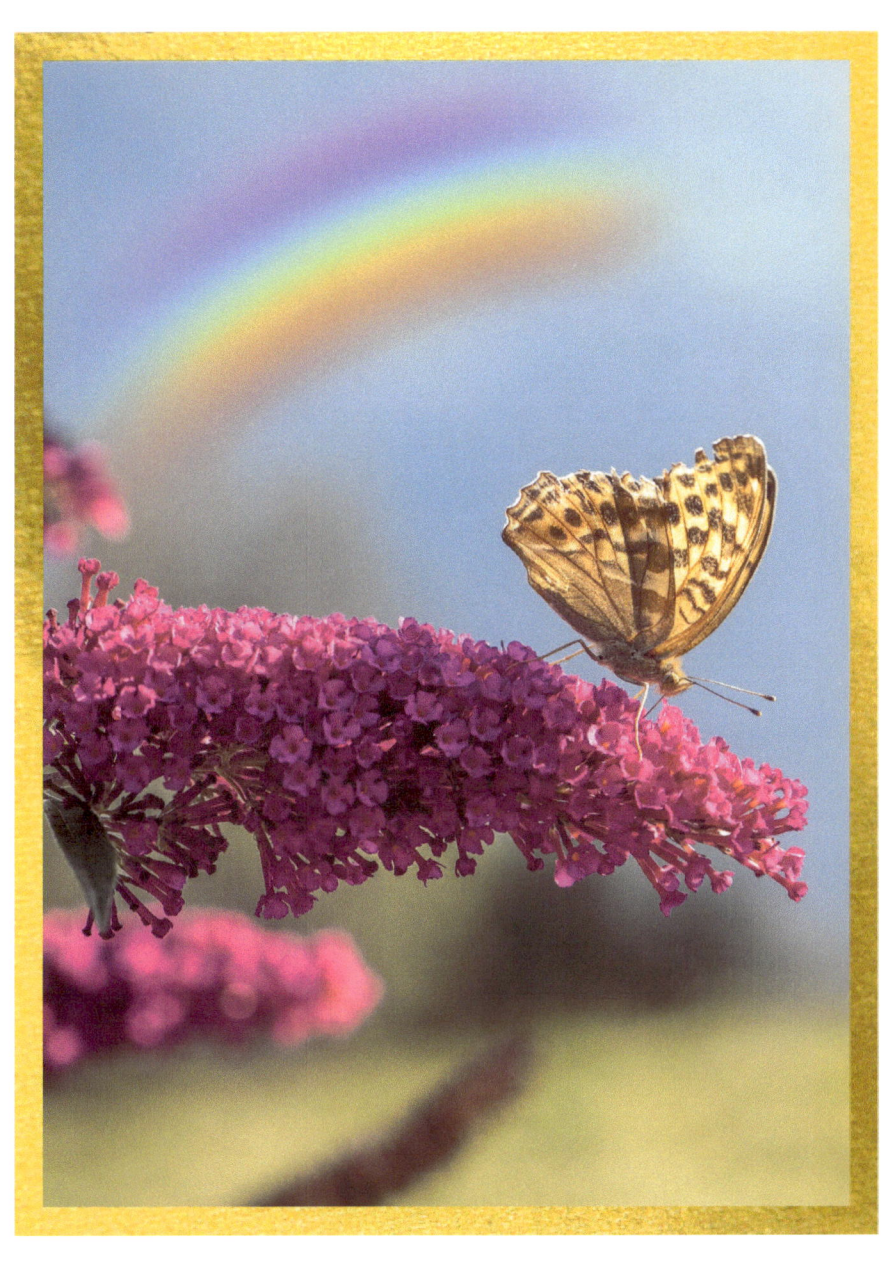

Nature never fails to amaze me

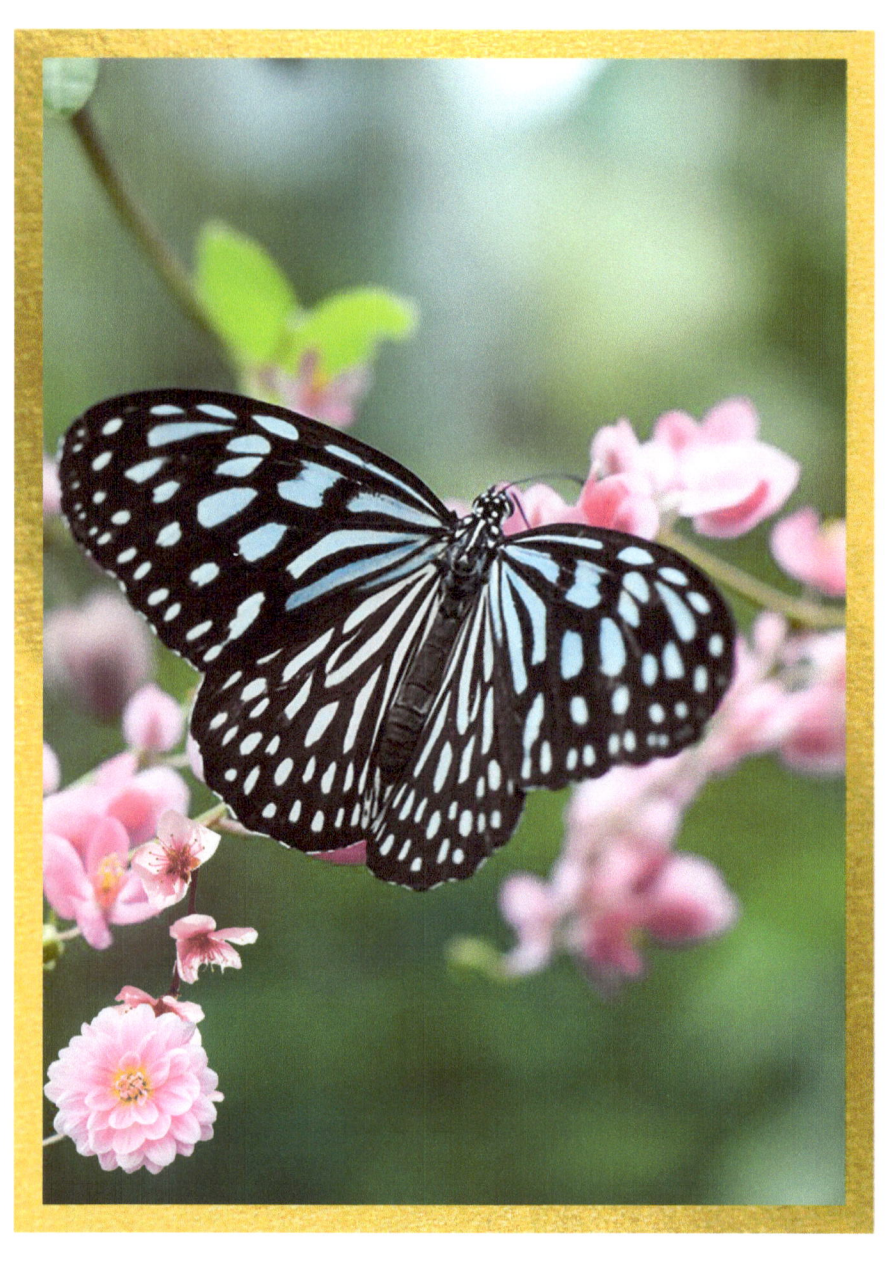

I'm a black beauty

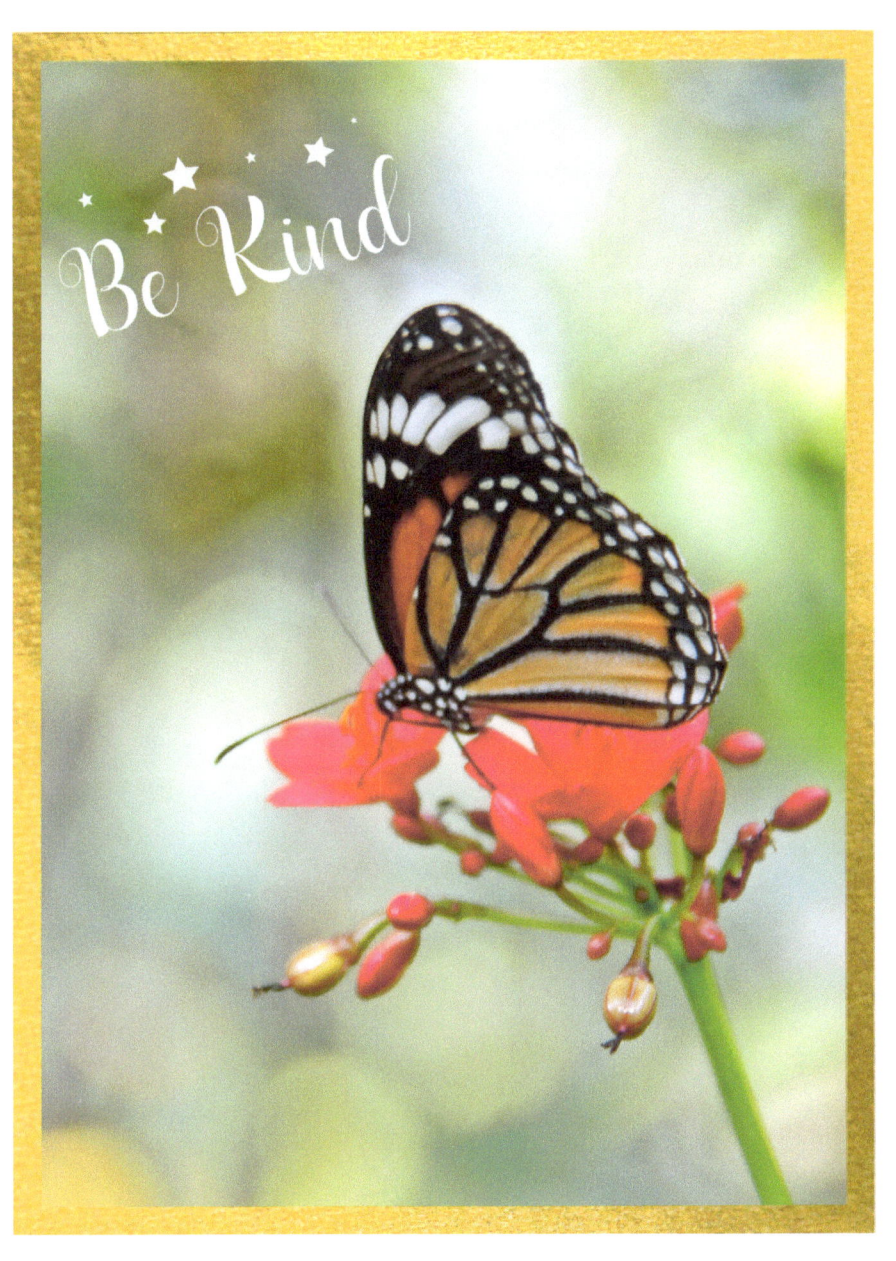

Rest & find peace

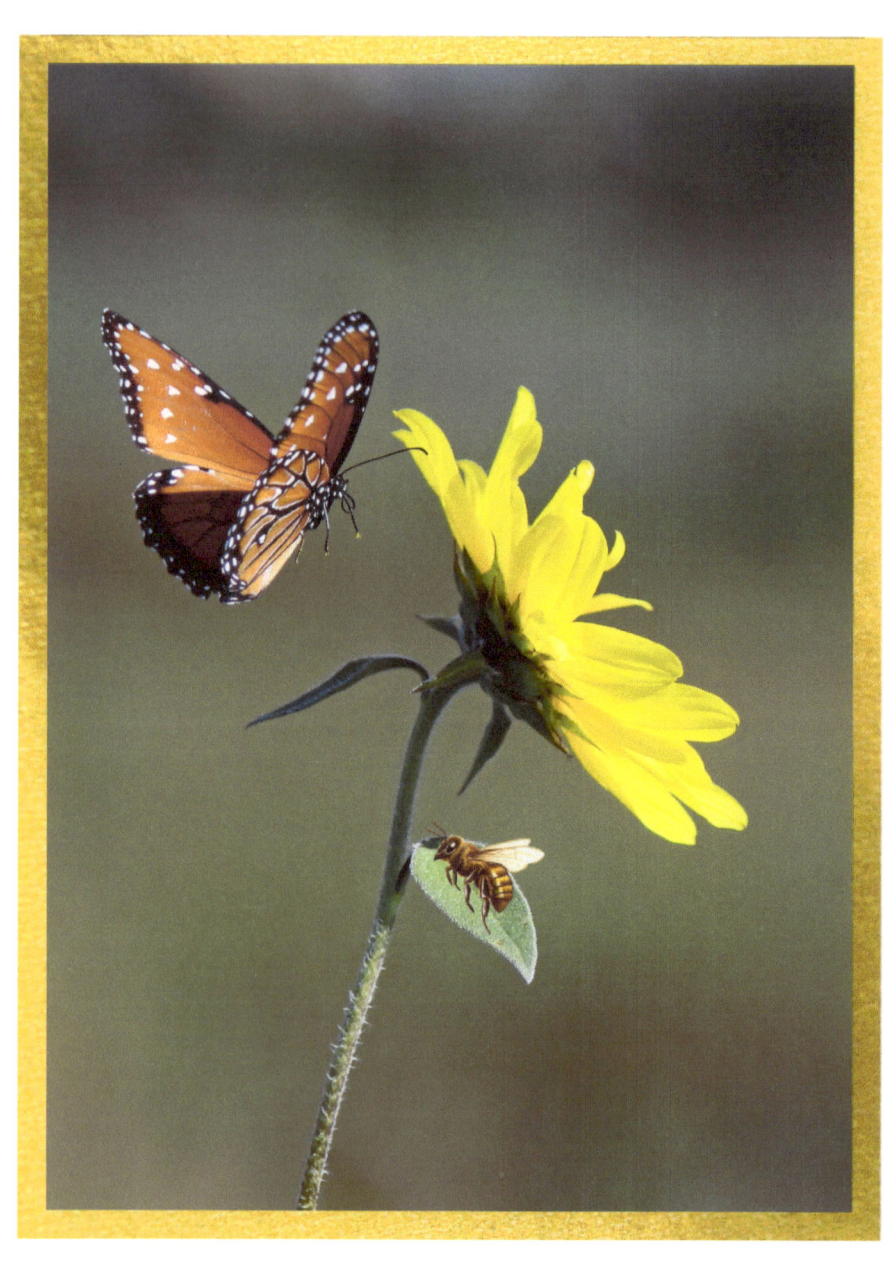

Spread your wings & be free!

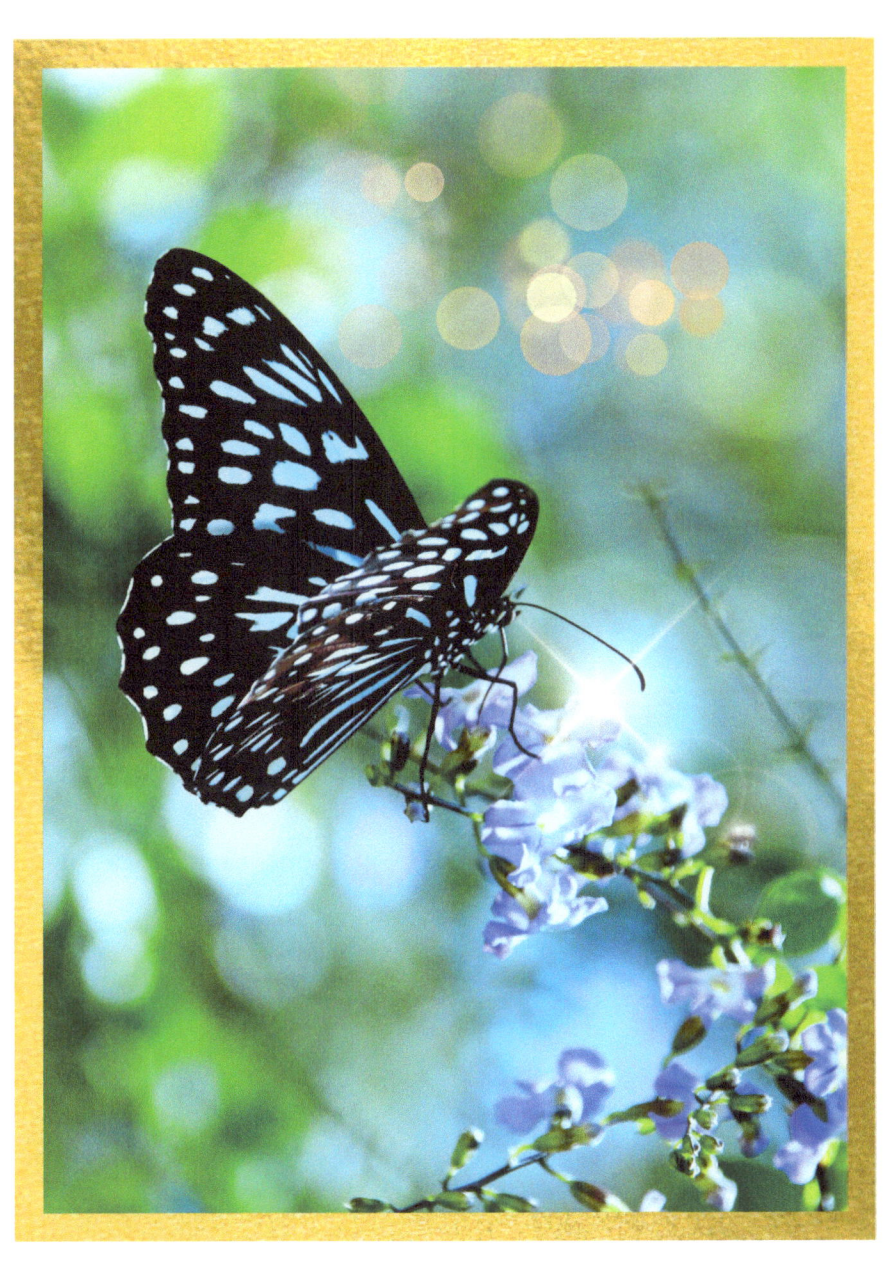

Patience is a virtue

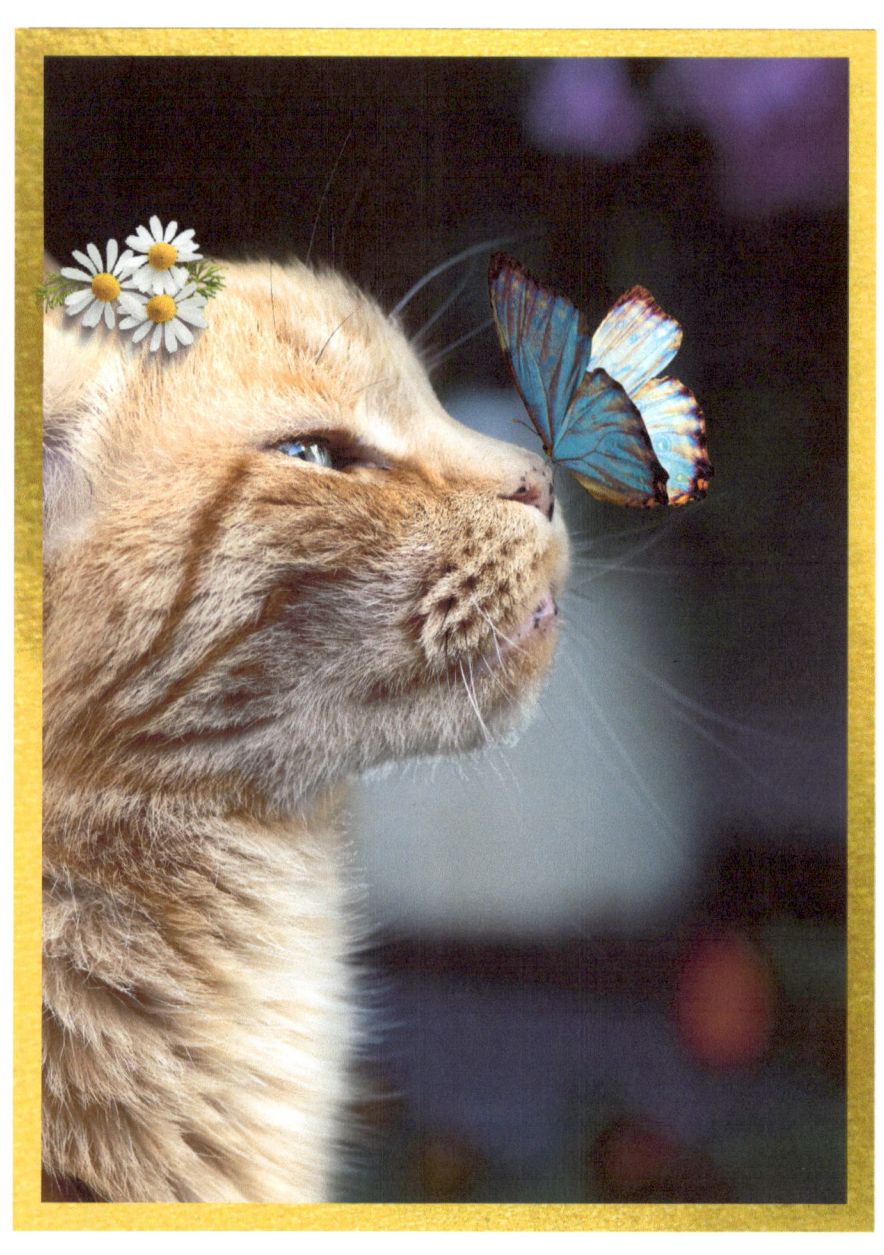

We are friends, aren't we?

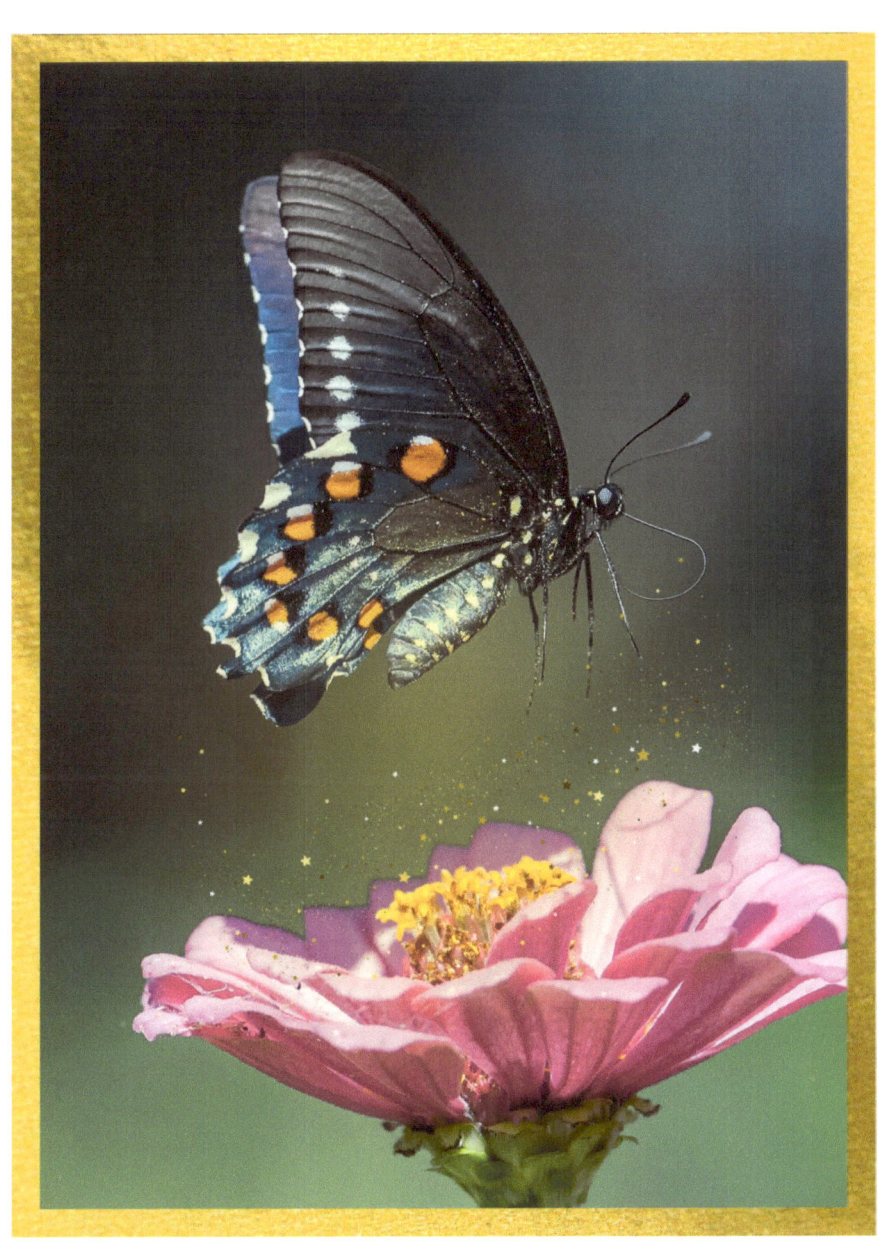

Give me a smile, baby

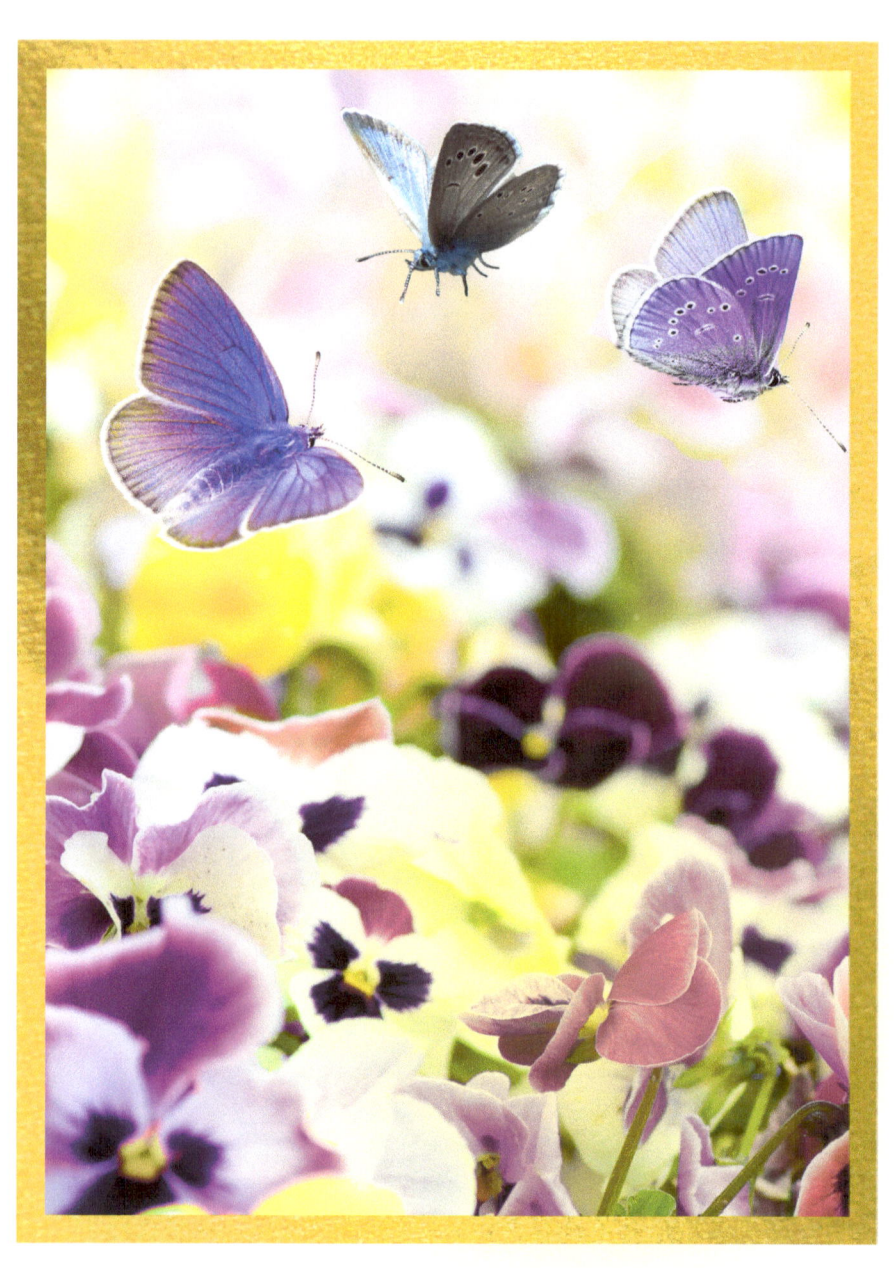

Isn't this a perfect?

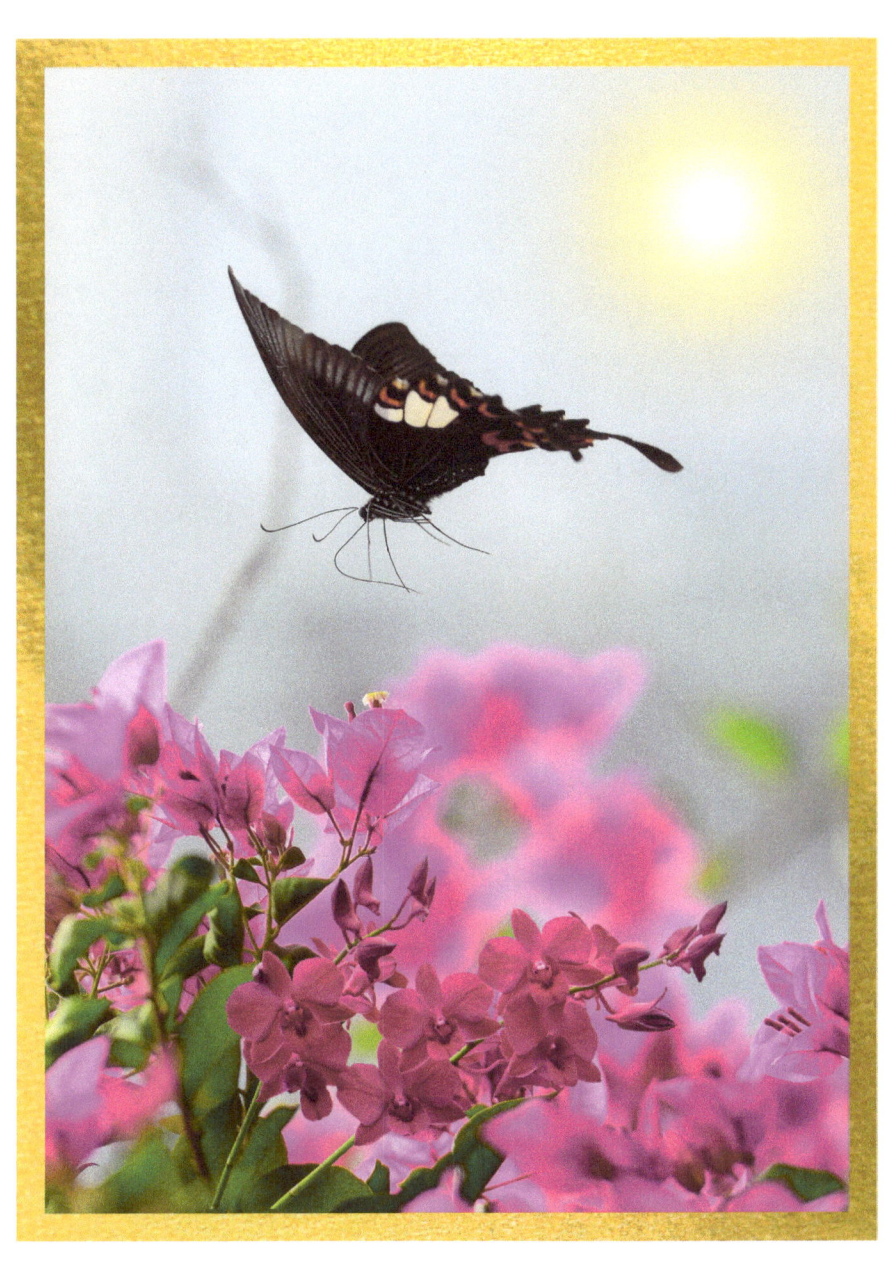

I'll love to give it a kiss

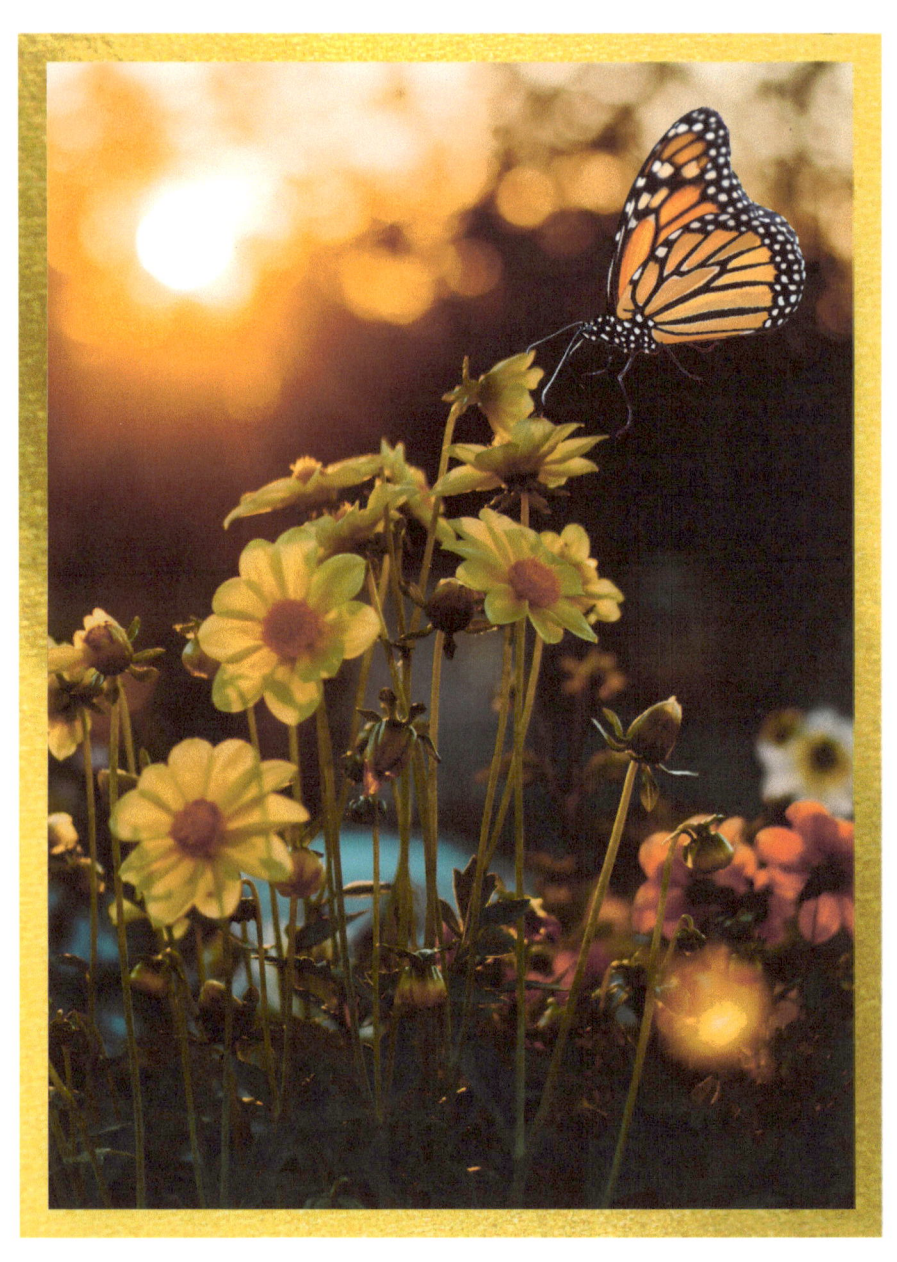

Good evening! I wish you well.

Dear Friend,

We hope you thoroughly enjoyed this picture book of beautiful butterflies.

As a way of saying thank you for your support of our creation, we would love to send you a bonus gift which you will love!

You can either click on this link:

https://prodigious-thinker-229.ck.page/22314404e3

Or scan the QR code below to claim your free gift.

We would appreciate if you can leave us a review to encourage our work.

Yours Sincerely,
Dana Wee & Team